The Low-FODMAP Kitchen

Easy and Tasty Recipes for a Healthier Gut

DAPHNE ADAMS

© Copyright 2024 Daphne Adams
All rights reserved.

The content contained within this book may not be reproduced, duplicated, or transmitted without direct written permission from the author or the publisher.

Under no circumstances will any blame or legal responsibility be held against the publisher or author, for any damages, reparation, or monetary loss due to the information contained within this book, either directly or indirectly.

LEGAL NOTICE:

This book is copyright-protected. It is only for personal use. You cannot amend, distribute, sell, use, quote, or paraphrase any part, or the content within this book, without the written consent of the author or publisher.

DISCLAIMER NOTICE:

Please note the information contained within this document is for educational and entertainment purposes only. All effort has been executed to present accurate, up-to-date, reliable, and complete information. No warranties of any kind are declared or implied. Readers acknowledge that the author is not engaged in the rendering of legal, financial, medical, or professional advice. The content within this book has been derived from various sources. Please consult a licensed professional before attempting any techniques outlined in this book.

By reading this document, the reader agrees that under no circumstances is the author responsible for any losses, direct or indirect, that are incurred as a result of the use of the information contained within this document, including but not limited to, errors, omissions, or inaccuracies.

TABLE OF CONTENTS

INTRODUCTION ... 6

CHAPTER 1: BREAKFAST ... 8

Sweet Potato Pancakes with Raspberries ... 8
Poached Egg Sandwich with Smoked Salmon ... 9
Poached Eggs with Lemon Hollandaise Sauce ... 10
Ham & Cheese Strata ... 11
Vegan French Toast ... 12
Carrot Cake Porridge ... 13
Scrambled Tofu ... 14
Tropical Millet Porridge ... 15
Spinach, Feta & Pine Nut Omelet ... 16
Quinoa Porridge with Banana & Yogurt ... 17
Ham, Cheese, and Spinach Breakfast Muffins ... 18
Shakshuka ... 19
Chia Seed Pudding ... 20
Baked Sweet Potatoes with Almond Butter ... 21
Gluten-Free Waffles with Strawberries ... 22
Protein Overnight Oats ... 23
Huevos Rancheros Hummus Toast ... 24
Peach and Raspberry Smoothie ... 25
Coconut Blueberry Smoothie ... 26
Coconut Lime Smoothie ... 27

CHAPTER 2: SNACKS ... 28

Pumpkin Spice Protein Balls ... 28
Salted Caramel Peanut Candy Bars ... 29
Muesli Bars ... 30
Savory Muffin ... 31
Peanut Butter Energy Bars ... 32
Mixed Berry & Yogurt Granola Bar ... 33

Spiced Molasses Cookies 34
Peanut Butter and Hemp Seed Protein Balls 35
Cranberry Orange Protein Balls 36
Fig and Date Energy Balls 37

CHAPTER 3: LUNCH 38

Quinoa Tabbouleh 38
Grilled Lamb Chops with Mint 39
Shrimp Saganaki 40
Mediterranean Chicken Skewers 41
Salmon with Dill and Lemon 43
Chicken Piccata 44
Greek-Style Meatballs 46
Chicken and Gnocchi Casserole 48
Warm Chicken and Roast Vegetable Salad 50
Asian-Inspired Quinoa Salad 52
Tandoori Chicken 53
Sheet Pan Greek Lemon Chicken and Potatoes 54
Low-FODMAP Vietnamese Pho 55
Low-FODMAP Japanese Chicken Katsu 56
Pork Lettuce Wraps 58
Beef Burger with Lactose-Free Cheese 59
Chicken Avocado Burger 60
Salmon Burger 61
Turkey Burger with Spinach 62
Veggie Burger (Quinoa & Carrot) 63

CHAPTER 4: DINNER 64

Salmon Bowls with Avocado and Carrot "Rice" 64
Grilled Shrimp with Lemon and Herbs 65
Mediterranean Baked Cod with Tomatoes and Olives 66
Mediterranean Salmon with Caper Relish 67
Garlic-Infused Olive Oil Shrimp and Spinach Sauté 68
Orange Ginger Grilled Chicken 69
Pumpkin Chicken Chili 70

Zucchini and Ground Turkey Skillet 71
One-Skillet Ground Turkey Thai Curry with Rice 72
Mongolian Turkey 73
Turkey Meatballs with Tomato Basil Sauce 74
Lemon Herb Turkey Cutlets with Roasted Vegetables 75
Turkey Stuffed Bell Peppers 76
Turkey Patties with Olive Tapenade 77
Basil Coconut Milk Ground Beef Skillet 78
Spiced Beef Patties with Cucumber Yogurt Sauce 80
Beef and Tomato Stir-Fry with Fresh Basil 81
Creamy Vegan Mushroom Soup 82
Shredded Brussels Sprout Salad with Roasted Sweet Potatoes 83
Vegan Mexican Black Bean and Sweet Potato Skillet 85

CHAPTER 5: DESSERT 86

Berry Frangipane Tart 86
Lemon & Blueberry Cheesecake Slice 87
Clafoutis Cake 88
Banana Bars 89
Lemon Cream Pie Bars 90
Tiramisu 91
Chocolate Truffles 93
Pineapple Upside-Down Cake 94
Chocolate Cake 95
Blueberry Cobbler 97

CHAPTER 6: PRACTICAL TIPS AND RECOMMENDATIONS 99

A guide to reading ingredients lists while on
a low-FODMAP diet 99
Eating out on a low-FODMAP diet 100
Traveling on a low-FODMAP diet 102
30-Day Low-FODMAP Diet Plan For IBS 103

INTRODUCTION

Irritable Bowel Syndrome (IBS) is a common condition affecting millions of people, characterized by symptoms such as bloating, abdominal pain, changes in bowel habits, and general digestive discomfort. Many people living with IBS seek effective ways to alleviate their symptoms, and a low-FODMAP diet has proven to be a beneficial approach. This cookbook offers a variety of dishes to support your health, allowing you to enjoy delicious meals without worrying about unpleasant side effects.

Essential Dietary Recommendations

A low-FODMAP diet was designed to reduce stress on the digestive system. FODMAPs are certain types of carbohydrates that can be poorly absorbed in the small intestine, leading to fermentation in the large intestine. This fermentation process can cause gas and increased liquid levels in the intestines, often leading to uncomfortable symptoms like bloating and diarrhea.

A Three-Phase Approach to Managing the Diet

1. **Elimination Phase:** During this initial stage, all high-FODMAP foods are removed from your diet. This helps to minimize symptoms and gain a clearer understanding of how your body reacts to different types of food. The elimination phase typically lasts between 4-6 weeks but consulting with a healthcare provider or dietitian is recommended for a personalized assessment.

2. **Reintroduction Phase:** After the elimination period, specific foods are gradually reintroduced to identify which ones trigger symptoms. This helps uncover your individual "triggers" and reduces unnecessary dietary restrictions.

3. **Personalization Phase:** In the final stage, a personalized eating plan is developed that excludes only those foods that cause discomfort, enabling you to enjoy a wide range of foods without fearing IBS symptoms.

Additional Ways to Support Your Health Beyond Diet

Beyond dietary adjustments, several other strategies can enhance the quality of life for those with IBS. Consider these tips:

- **Regular Physical Activity:** Moderate exercise supports healthy digestive function. Even simple activities like daily walks, yoga, or swimming can help reduce stress and improve digestion.

- **Keeping a Food Diary:** Recording what you eat and any symptoms you experience makes it easier to track which foods and situations trigger discomfort. This also helps you adhere to the diet more accurately and identify triggers more quickly.

- **Stress Reduction:** It's well-known that stress can exacerbate IBS symptoms. Mindfulness practices, meditation, and deep breathing can help manage stress and improve emotional well-being.

- **Staying Hydrated:** Water is essential for maintaining healthy bowel function, especially if you experience constipation. Aim to drink enough water each day to keep your body well-hydrated.

- **Following a Regular Eating Schedule:** Try to maintain a regular eating routine with smaller meal portions. This prevents overloading the digestive system and minimizes IBS symptoms.

Psychological Support

Mental health plays an important role in managing IBS. Healthcare providers often recommend Cognitive Behavioral Therapy (CBT) to help manage anxiety related to IBS and gain control over symptoms. Therapy and emotional support can help you cope with the condition and improve your quality of life.

Incorporating stress-reduction practices, such as yoga or meditation, can be particularly beneficial. These practices help you relax, reduce stress levels, and positively impact digestive health.

Talk to Your Doctor

A low-FODMAP diet, along with other recommendations, such as regular physical activity and stress management, can significantly relieve IBS symptoms. However, it's important to remember that making changes to your diet on your own may not always be safe. It's advisable to consult with a doctor or qualified dietitian before making major lifestyle or dietary changes.

In this cookbook, you'll find recipes and tips designed to improve your well-being and add variety to your meals, despite the restrictions that come with IBS.

CHAPTER 1: BREAKFASTS
Sweet Potato Pancakes with Raspberries

Serves: 2
Prep: 10 minutes | **Cook:** 15 minutes

Nutrition:

Cal 320 | **Fat** 12g
Carb 50g | **Protein** 8g

Ingredients:

For the Pancakes:
- ½cup cooked and mashed sweet potato (ensure it's smooth)
- ½cup gluten-free all-purpose flour
- ¼tsp baking powder
- 1 egg
- ½cup lactose-free milk (or almond milk)
- 1tbsp maple syrup
- ½tsp vanilla extract
- ¼tsp cinnamon
- A pinch of salt
- 1tbsp lactose-free butter or oil for cooking

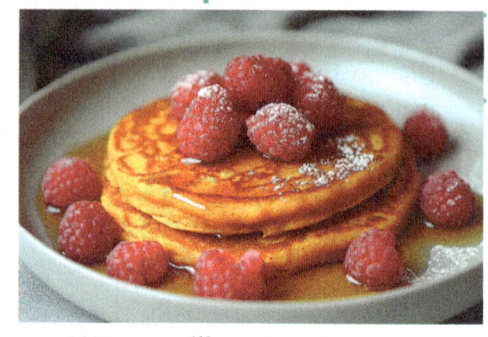

For the Topping:
- ½cup fresh raspberries
- 2tbsp maple syrup (optional)
- Lactose-free whipped cream (optional)

Instructions:

1. In a medium bowl, whisk together the mashed sweet potato, egg, lactose-free milk, vanilla extract, and maple syrup.
2. In another bowl, mix the gluten-free flour, baking powder, cinnamon, and a pinch of salt.
3. Gradually add the dry ingredients to the wet ingredients, stirring until combined and smooth.
4. Heat a non-stick skillet over medium heat and add a little lactose-free butter or oil.
5. Pour about ¼cup of the batter onto the skillet for each pancake. Cook for 2-3 minutes on each side, or until bubbles form on the surface and the pancakes are golden brown.
6. Stack the pancakes on a plate, top with fresh raspberries, and drizzle with maple syrup if desired.
7. Optionally, add a dollop of lactose-free whipped cream for extra indulgence.

Chapter 1: Breakfasts

Poached Egg Sandwich with Smoked Salmon

Serves: 2
Prep: 10 minutes | **Cook:** 10 minutes

Nutrition:

Cal 350 | **Fat** 18g
Carb 25g | **Protein** 20g

Ingredients:

For the Sandwich:
- 2 eggs (for poaching)
- 2 slices gluten-free bread
- 3.5oz smoked salmon (ensure no added high-FODMAP ingredients)
- ½ ripe avocado, mashed (optional, moderate FODMAP in large amounts)
- Fresh dill or chives (optional, for garnish)
- Salt and pepper to taste

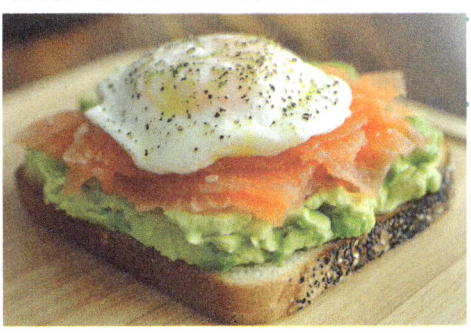

For the Poached Eggs:
- 2cups water
- 1tbsp white vinegar (optional, helps eggs set while poaching)

Instructions:

1. In a small saucepan, bring water and vinegar to a gentle simmer.
2. Crack one egg into a small bowl. Stir the simmering water to create a gentle whirlpool, then carefully slide the egg into the center. Cook for 3-4 minutes, or until the whites are set but the yolk remains runny.
3. Remove with a slotted spoon and place on a plate. Repeat with the second egg.
4. While the eggs are poaching, toast the gluten-free bread slices to your desired crispness.
5. On each slice of toasted gluten-free bread, spread the mashed avocado (optional) as a base layer. Top with the smoked salmon, followed by the poached egg.
6. Season with salt and pepper to taste. Garnish with fresh dill or chives, if desired.
7. Serve the sandwiches immediately, while the eggs and toast are still warm.

Poached Eggs with Lemon Hollandaise Sauce

Serves: 2
Prep: 10 minutes | **Cook:** 10 minutes

Nutrition:

Cal 289 | **Fat** 24g
Carb 2g | **Protein** 14g

Ingredients:

Eggs:
- 1tbsp white vinegar
- 4 eggs
- Buttered low-FODMAP or gluten-free toast, to serve
- Handful of mixed lettuce leaves, to serve
- A few grinds of salt and pepper

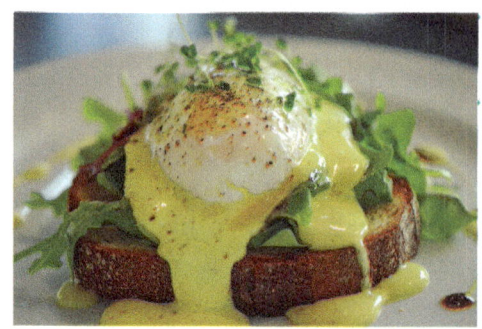

Lemon Hollandaise Sauce:
- 1½tbsp lemon juice
- 2 egg yolks
- A pinch of white sugar
- A pinch of rock salt
- Black pepper, to taste
- 2tbsp dairy-free spread or butter

Instructions:

1. Fill a deep-frying pan with about 1¼inches of water and add the vinegar. Bring the water to a rolling boil, then turn it down to a gentle simmer.
2. Take an egg and crack it into a small sieve (this removes any loose egg white and gives you a pretty poached egg), then carefully pour it into a small bowl.
3. Stir the water until it swirls and carefully pour the whole egg into the pan. Repeat for each egg.
4. Cook each egg for about 2 minutes for a soft egg or 4 minutes for a firmer egg, then scoop out and place on a paper towel to drain.
5. Make the hollandaise sauce while the eggs cook. Whisk the lemon juice, egg yolks, sugar, salt, and black pepper together in a small bowl until smooth. Melt the dairy-free spread or butter in the microwave and slowly whisk into the mixture.
6. Heat the hollandaise sauce in the microwave for 15 seconds, whisk, and then heat in 10-second bursts (you might need to do this four or five times), whisking each time to remove the skin that forms on the sides of the bowl. Repeat until thick.
7. Serve the poached eggs on buttered toast with mixed lettuce leaves. Drizzle with hollandaise sauce and season with salt and pepper to taste.

Chapter 1: Breakfasts

Ham & Cheese Strata

Serves: 2
Prep: 10 minutes | **Cook:** 35 minutes

Nutrition:

Cal 163 | **Fat** 10g
Carb 18g | **Protein** 12g

Ingredients:

- 2 slices of gluten-free bread, cut into cubes
- ½cup diced ham (ensure no high-FODMAP ingredients like garlic or onion)
- ½cup lactose-free shredded cheddar cheese
- 2 large eggs
- ½cup lactose-free milk
- ½tsp Dijon mustard (optional)
- Salt and pepper to taste
- ¼tsp dried thyme or fresh herbs for garnish (optional)

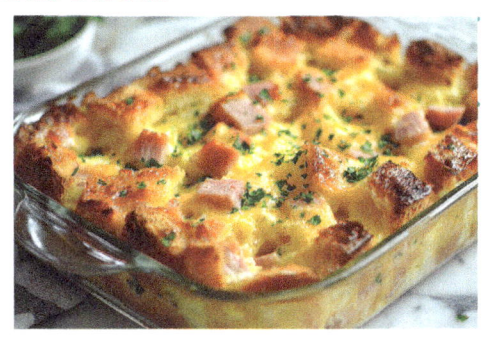

Instructions:

1. Preheat your oven to 350°F (180°C). Lightly grease a small baking dish or two individual ramekins.
2. In the baking dish, lay half of the cubed gluten-free bread, followed by half of the diced ham and shredded cheese.
3. Repeat with the remaining bread, ham, and cheese.
4. In a mixing bowl, whisk together the eggs, lactose-free milk, Dijon mustard (if using), salt, and pepper.
5. Pour the egg mixture evenly over the bread, ham, and cheese layers, pressing down lightly to ensure the bread soaks up the liquid.
6. Let the mixture sit for 5-10 minutes to allow the bread to absorb the liquid fully.
7. Bake in the preheated oven for 30-35 minutes, or until the top is golden and the center is set. If the top browns too quickly, cover with aluminum foil and continue baking until done.
8. Remove from the oven and allow it to cool for a few minutes before serving.
9. Garnish with fresh herbs, if desired.

Vegan French Toast

Serves: 2
Prep: 5 minutes | **Cook:** 5 minutes

Nutrition:

Cal 324 | **Fat** 11g
Carb 33g | **Protein** 18g

Ingredients:

- ½ cup soy milk (made with soy protein)
- 5oz firm tofu
- 1tsp vanilla extract
- 2tsp cinnamon
- 2tsp nutmeg
- 4 slices of gluten-free bread or spelt sourdough bread
- 2tsp of oil for cooking or cooking oil spray
- Maple syrup to serve

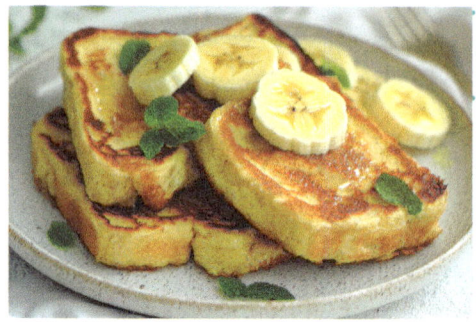

Instructions:

1. Add the tofu, soy milk, vanilla extract, cinnamon, and nutmeg to a blender and process until well combined. If you don't have a blender, just give it a good whisk in a small bowl.
2. Pour the wet mix into a shallow dish and add the bread. Leave the bread to soak for a minute or so, then flip it over to make sure the other side of the bread is coated.
3. Heat a non-stick frying pan over medium-high heat and add oil. When the oil is hot, add the bread to the frying pan. Cook on one side for a few minutes until golden brown, then flip the bread over and cook until the other side is golden brown.
4. Serve on a plate and top with maple syrup.

Topping suggestions:

- Your favorite low-FODMAP fruits like bananas or blueberries
- Lactose-free yogurt.

Chapter 1: Breakfasts

Carrot Cake Porridge

Serves: 2
Prep: 5 minutes | **Cook:** 20 minutes

Nutrition:

Cal 290 | **Fat** 14g
Carb 30g | **Protein** 10g

Ingredients:

- ½cup oats
- 1½cups water
- 1 medium carrot, grated
- ½tsp cinnamon
- ½tbsp linseeds (flaxseeds)
- 2tbsp raisins or dried cranberries
- 2tbsp walnuts (or other low-FODMAP nuts you like)
- ¼cup milk of your choice
- 2tbsp hemp seeds (optional)
- Maple syrup to serve

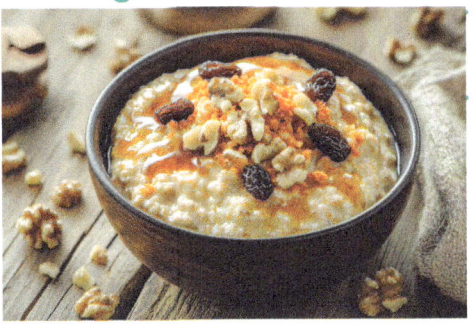

Instructions:

1. In a medium pot, add the oats and water, stirring with a wooden spoon over medium heat.
2. When the oats just come to a boil, turn the heat down and add the carrots and cinnamon, stirring.
3. When the porridge has cooked to your liking, about 10-12 minutes total, take off the heat and stir in the linseeds (flaxseeds), dried fruit, and nuts.
4. Serve into 2 bowls and top with the milk, maple syrup and to boost your protein, 1tbsp of hemp seeds.

Scrambled Tofu

Serves: 2
Prep: 5 minutes | **Cook:** 5 minutes

Nutrition:

Cal 229 | **Fat** 17g
Carb 3g | **Protein** 13g

Ingredients:

- 7oz firm tofu
- ½cup water
- 2tsp soy sauce
- ½tsp ground turmeric*
- 1cup diced or grated carrot and zucchini
- Cooking oil for frying or cooking oil spray

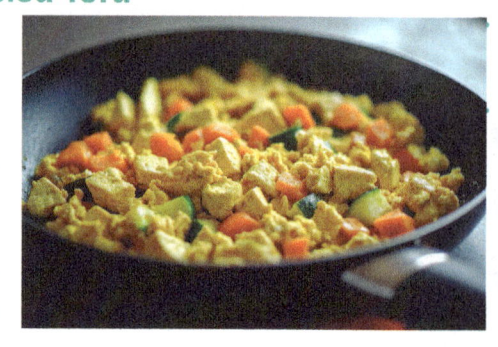

*This will give the tofu a yellow color which will make it resemble scrambled eggs

Instructions:

1. Place the water, soy sauce, and turmeric in a bowl and mix well.
2. Crumble the tofu into the bowl using your fingers and add the vegetables.
3. Heat the oil in a small frying pan over medium heat and add the contents of the bowl. Gently fry until golden brown (about 5 minutes).
4. Serve with cooked rice or sourdough spelt bread.

Chapter 1: Breakfasts

Tropical Millet Porridge

Serves: 2
Prep: 5 minutes | **Cook:** 30 minutes

Nutrition:

Cal 465 | **Fat** 19g
Carb 58g | **Protein** 12g

Ingredients:

- ⅔ cup hulled millet seed
- 1⅓ cups water (boiling)
- Pinch of salt
- ⅓ cup soy protein milk (lactose-free milk or almond milk)
- 2tbsp dried shredded coconut
- 1.75oz strawberries
- 2oz banana
- Pinch of cinnamon
- 2tsp maple syrup

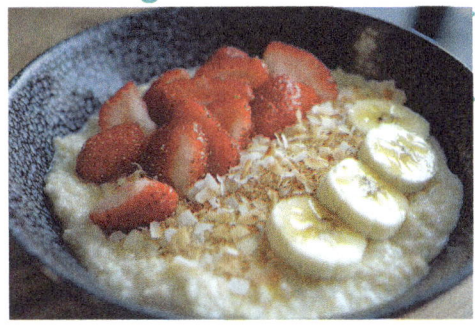

Instructions:

1. Toast the millet seed in a saucepan over medium high heat for about 2-3 minutes until it starts to go golden. Add the boiling water and a pinch of salt. Then cover and simmer on the lowest heat setting for 15 to 20 minutes, until most of the water absorbs and the millet is soft. Allow to stand for 5 minutes.
2. Peel and slice the banana and cut the strawberries into quarters.
3. Once the millet is cooked, you can then stir through your choice of low-FODMAP milk until it is creamy (add more low-FODMAP milk if needed). Stir through the shredded coconut and a few pinches of cinnamon. Divide between two bowls and top with the strawberries, banana and a drizzle of pure maple syrup.

Notes for cooking millet the night before:

- Complete step one in the method. Store the millet in an airtight container in the refrigerator. In the morning, break up the millet using a fork. Transfer to bowls and add your low-FODMAP milk. Heat in the microwave until warm. Then stir through the cinnamon, shredded coconut, and low-FODMAP fruit. Drizzle with maple syrup.

Spinach, Feta & Pine Nut Omelet

Serves: 2
Prep: 5 minutes | **Cook:** 5 minutes

Nutrition:

Cal 337 | **Fat** 26g
Carb 3g | **Protein** 24g

Ingredients:

- 4 large eggs
- 2tbsp milk (lactose-free if required)
- Pinch of pepper, to taste
- 2tsp butter
- 2cups of baby spinach
- ½cup crumbled feta cheese
- 2tbsp toasted pine nuts

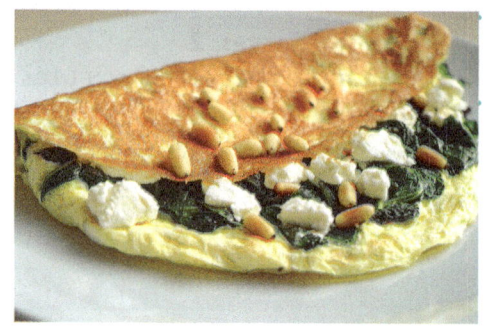

Instructions:

1. Wilt the spinach in a lightly oiled pan and fold through the feta to warm. Set aside.
2. Lightly whisk the eggs with milk and a pinch of pepper.
3. In a non-stick fry pan melt the butter over a moderate heat while swirling over the surface until it starts to sizzle.
4. Pour in the egg mix and swirl the pan ensuring a thin, round omelet is formed. Briefly cover with a tight fitting lid so the surface egg is almost cooked.
5. Spoon the warmed filling on half the omelet and again cover for about 20 seconds. Remove the lid and sprinkle with pine nuts.
6. Tip the pan towards the serving plate and fold the omelet in half to encase the filling.
7. Slip the omelet onto the plate and serve with any low-FODMAP toasted bread.

Note:

- For a nut-free option replace pine nuts with toasted sunflower seeds.

Chapter 1: Breakfasts

Quinoa Porridge with Banana & Yogurt

Serves: 2
Prep: 5 minutes | **Cook:** 10 minutes

Nutrition:

Cal 470 | **Fat** 9g
Carb 77g | **Protein** 20g

Ingredients:

- 1cup of water
- 2cups of lactose-free milk (or low-fat alternative)
- 3.5oz quinoa flakes
- 2/3 ripe banana (or 2/3 unripe, slightly green banana)
- 3.5oz lactose-free yogurt (or plain low-fat Greek yogurt)
- 2tsp maple syrup
- Sprinkle of cinnamon (optional)

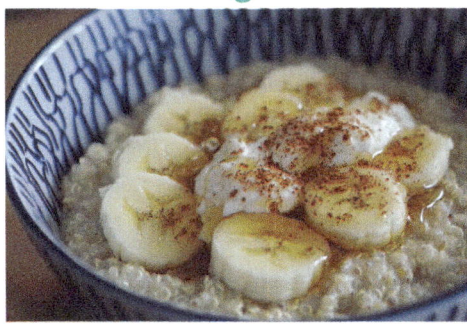

Instructions:

1. In a small saucepan, bring the water and half of the milk to the boil on the stove, then add your quinoa flakes. Turn the heat down to low and allow simmering for approximately 5 minutes.
2. Meanwhile, slice the banana and set it aside.
3. When the quinoa reaches a thickened consistency, pour in a bowl and top off with the remaining milk. Add the yogurt and banana with a drizzle of maple syrup. Sprinkle some cinnamon over the quinoa porridge for extra flavor.

Ham, Cheese, and Spinach Breakfast Muffins

Serves: 6 | **Prep:** 10 minutes
Cook: 20-25 minutes

Nutrition:

Cal 316 | **Fat** 12g
Carb 36g | **Protein** 17g

Ingredients:

- 1½ cups corn (maize) flour
- ½ cup oat bran
- 2½ tsp baking powder
- ½ tsp xanthan gum
- ⅔ cup cream (thickened or pouring ~35% fat)
- ½ cup low-fat milk (use lactose-free if required). A little extra if required
- 2 large eggs
- 1 cup diced, lean good-quality ham
- ½ cup chives, chopped
- ¾ cup low-fat, grated cheddar cheese
- 1¼ cup baby spinach, roughly chopped
- Olive oil spray for muffin cases
- ⅓ cup grated, low-fat cheddar cheese
- ½ tsp smoked paprika

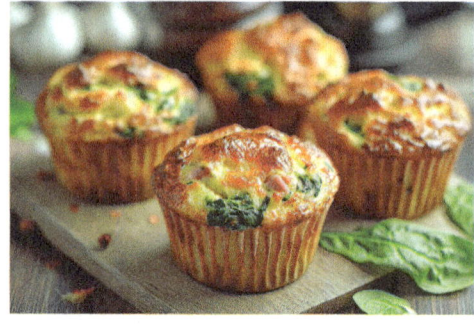

Instructions:

1. Preheat oven to 160°C/320°F (180°C/356°F if not fan-forced) and on a lower shelf of the oven, half-fill a baking tray with boiling water.
2. Sift flour, baking powder, and xanthan gum into a large bowl then stir through the bran.
3. In a separate bowl, whisk eggs with the cream and milk. Stir in ham, chives, spinach, and cheese.
4. Make a well in the flour mix and fold the wet mix into the dry ingredients. You may have to add more milk to achieve dough that is slightly sloppy but not too wet.
5. Place large muffin cases in a muffin tray and spray well with olive oil.
6. Fill muffin cases (see tip below) and tap down the top surface with a wet finger.
7. Sprinkle the top of each muffin with grated cheese, then paprika.
8. Bake for about 20 to 25 minutes until golden brown (an inserted skewer should be clean when removed).

Chapter 1: Breakfasts

Shakshuka

Serves: 2
Prep: 10 minutes | **Cook:** 20 minute

Nutrition:

Cal 220 | **Fat** 14g
Carb 18g | **Protein** 12g

Ingredients:

- 1tbsp garlic infused olive oil
- ½ medium zucchini
- ½ bunch kale
- ¼tsp paprika
- ¼tsp cumin
- ⅛tsp cinnamon
- ½can fire roasted tomatoes or plain canned tomatoes
- 2tbsp tomato paste
- 2tbsp low-FODMAP vegan broth; mixed into the tomato paste
- 1tbsp water
- 2 large eggs
- ¼tsp each of salt and pepper, plus to taste
- Fresh cilantro, chopped for garnish
- Feta or goat cheese, crumbled (optional, omit for dairy-free)
- Sliced avocado, or crusty gluten-free bread for serving

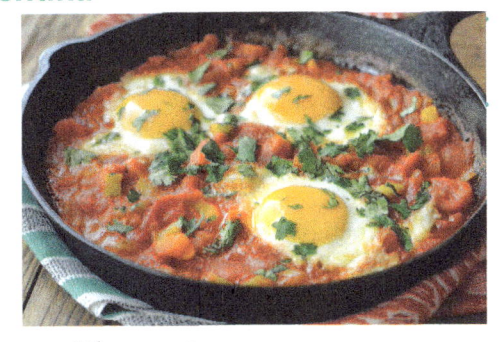

Instructions:

1. Heat infused oil in a large sauté pan over medium heat. Add the chopped zucchini and cook until soft, about 3-5 minutes.
2. Add the kale, and sprinkle with ½tsp salt and pepper. Stir fry until wilted, covering if necessary.
3. Pour the can of fire roasted tomatoes and juice into the pan, then add the tomato paste, broth, and then use the 2tbsp water to rinse the can and add to skillet. Sprinkle with all the spices and stir well. Season with additional salt and pepper, or additional spices to taste.
4. Allow the sauce to simmer, then use a large spoon to make small wells in the sauce and crack the eggs into each well.
5. Cover the pan and cook for 6-10 minutes, or until the eggs are done to your liking.
6. Garnish with chopped cilantro and optional cheese.

Chia Seed Pudding

Serves: 2 | **Prep:** 5 minutes
Cook: chill for 4 hours or overnight

Nutrition:

Cal 320 | **Fat** 15g
Carb 35g | **Protein** 12g

Ingredients:

- 4tbsp chia seeds
- 1cup lactose-free milk
- 1tsp vanilla extract
- 1tbsp maple syrup
- Fresh berries for topping

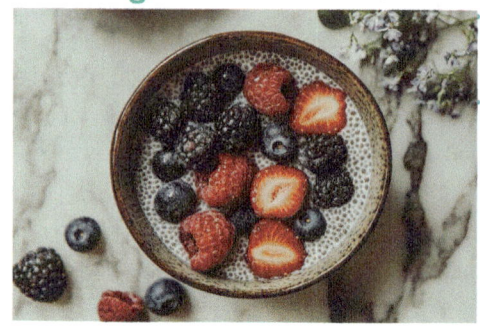

Instructions:

1. Mix chia seeds, milk, vanilla extract, and maple syrup in a bowl.
2. Stir well and refrigerate for at least 4 hours or overnight.
3. Serve with fresh berries on top.

Chapter 1: Breakfasts

Baked Sweet Potatoes with Almond Butter

Serves: 2
Prep: 5 minutes | **Cook:** 45 minutes

Nutrition:

Cal 280 | **Fat** 12g
Carb 40g | **Protein** 5g

Ingredients:

- 2 medium sweet potatoes
- 2tbsp almond butter
- 1tsp ground cinnamon
- 1tsp maple syrup (optional)
- A pinch of sea salt

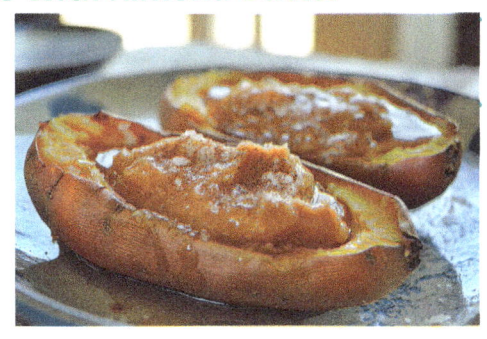

Instructions:

1. Preheat your oven to 400°F (200°C). Line a baking sheet with parchment paper.
2. Wash and scrub the sweet potatoes. Pierce each sweet potato several times with a fork to allow steam to escape.
3. Place the sweet potatoes on the prepared baking sheet and bake for 40-45 minutes, or until they are tender when pierced with a fork.
4. Once baked, cut the sweet potatoes open lengthwise.
5. Spread 1tbsp of almond butter on each sweet potato.
6. Sprinkle with ground cinnamon, drizzle with maple syrup (if using), and add a pinch of sea salt for a touch of flavor.
7. Serve hot as a delicious, filling, and nutritious low-FODMAP breakfast or snack.

Gluten-Free Waffles with Strawberries

Serves: 2
Prep: 10 minutes | **Cook:** 10 minute

Nutrition:

Cal 270 | **Fat** 12g
Carb 45g | **Protein** 7g

Ingredients:

For the Waffles:
- 1cup gluten-free all-purpose flour
- 1tbsp granulated sugar
- 1tsp baking powder
- ¼tsp salt
- 1 egg
- ½cup lactose-free milk (or almond milk)
- 1tbsp lactose-free butter or coconut oil, melted
- ½tsp vanilla extract

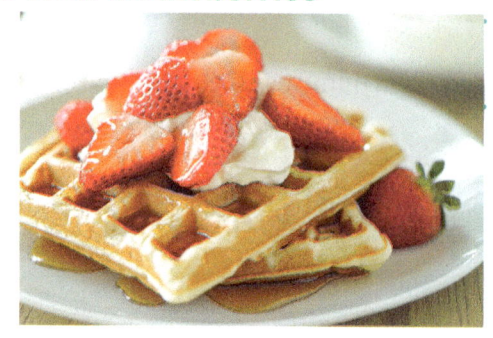

For the Topping:
- ½cup fresh strawberries, sliced
- 1tbsp maple syrup or honey (optional)
- Whipped lactose-free cream (optional)

Instructions:

1. Plug in your waffle iron and let it heat up according to the manufacturer's instructions.
2. In a medium bowl, whisk together the gluten-free flour, sugar, baking powder, and salt.
3. In another bowl, whisk the egg, lactose-free milk, melted butter (or coconut oil), and vanilla extract until combined.
4. Gradually add the wet ingredients to the dry ingredients, stirring until just combined. The batter should be smooth but avoid over-mixing.
5. Lightly grease the waffle iron with a bit of cooking spray or melted butter.
6. Pour about ¼ to 1/3cup of batter into the center of the waffle iron (amount depends on the size of your waffle iron) and close the lid.
7. Cook for 3-4 minutes, or until the waffles are golden and crisp.
8. While the waffles cook, wash and slice the strawberries. Optionally, drizzle with maple syrup or honey for extra sweetness.
9. Place the freshly cooked waffles on a plate. Top with sliced strawberries and, if desired, a dollop of lactose-free whipped cream.

Chapter 1: Breakfasts

Protein Overnight Oats

Serves: 2 | **Prep:** 5 minutes
Chill Time: 6-8 hours (overnight)

Nutrition:

Cal 362 | **Fat** 9g
Carb 51g | **Protein** 22g

Ingredients:

- 1cup gluten-free sprouted oats
- ½cup lactose-free non-fat Greek yogurt
- ½cup almond milk
- 1tbsp chia seeds (optional, for added fiber and texture)
- 1 scoop low-FODMAP vanilla protein powder
- 1tbsp maple syrup (optional, for sweetness)
- ½tsp vanilla extract
- Fresh blueberries or strawberries for topping (optional)

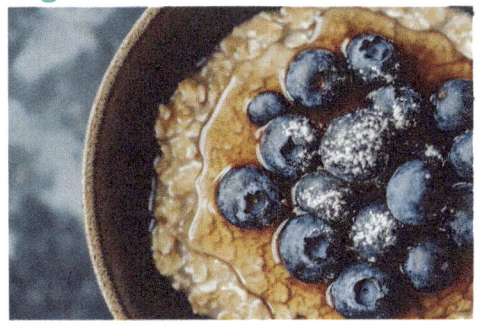

Instructions:

1. In a medium bowl or two individual jars, combine the gluten-free sprouted oats, lactose-free Greek yogurt, almond milk, chia seeds (if using), vanilla protein powder, and vanilla extract.
2. Stir well to ensure everything is mixed evenly.
3. Add 1 tablespoon of maple syrup if you'd like additional sweetness.
4. Cover the bowl or jars and refrigerate for at least 6-8 hours, or overnight, to allow the oats to soften and absorb the liquid.
5. In the morning, give the oats a good stir, and top with fresh berries, if desired.

Huevos Rancheros Hummus Toast

Serves: 2
Prep: 10 minutes | **Cook:** 15 minutes

Nutrition:

Cal 350 | **Fat** 18g
Carb 35g | **Protein** 15g

Ingredients:

- 4 slices gluten-free bread
- 2 large eggs
- ½cup low-FODMAP hummus (store-bought or homemade using garlic-infused oil)
- ½cup diced tomatoes (low-FODMAP serving size)
- ¼cup chopped green tops of scallions (green parts only)
- ¼tsp smoked paprika
- ¼tsp cumin
- 1tbsp olive oil
- 1tbsp fresh cilantro, chopped (optional for garnish)
- Salt and pepper to taste
- ¼ avocado (optional for topping; note: avocado is low-FODMAP in small servings)

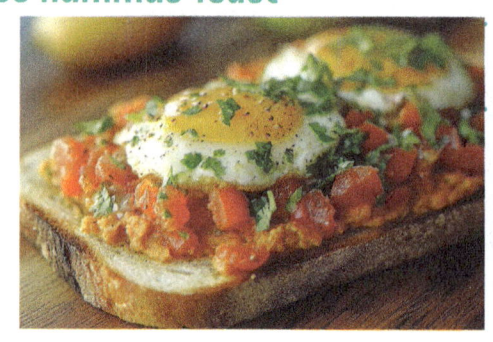

Instructions:

1. Toast the gluten-free bread slices to your desired crispness and set aside.
2. In a skillet, heat the olive oil over medium heat.
3. Add the diced tomatoes, green scallions (green parts only), smoked paprika, and cumin. Cook for 3-4 minutes until the tomatoes soften and the flavors combine. Season with salt and pepper to taste.
4. In the same skillet, push the tomato mixture to the side and crack two eggs into the skillet. Fry the eggs to your preferred doneness (sunny-side-up is traditional for huevos rancheros).
5. Spread an even layer of low-FODMAP hummus on each slice of toasted gluten-free bread.
6. Spoon the tomato mixture evenly on top of the hummus.
7. Top each toast with a fried egg.
8. Add thin slices of avocado (within the low-FODMAP limit) and fresh cilantro on top for extra flavor.

Chapter 1: Breakfasts

Peach and Raspberry Smoothie

Serves: 1 | **Prep:** 5 minutes
Cook: No cooking required

Nutrition:

Cal 180 | **Fat** 5g
Carb 30g | **Protein** 8g

Ingredients:

- ½ cup frozen or fresh peaches, sliced
- ½ cup raspberries (fresh or frozen)
- ½ cup lactose-free yogurt
- ½ cup lactose-free milk (or almond milk for a dairy-free option)
- 1 tsp honey or maple syrup (optional, for added sweetness)
- ¼ cup ice cubes (optional, for a thicker texture)

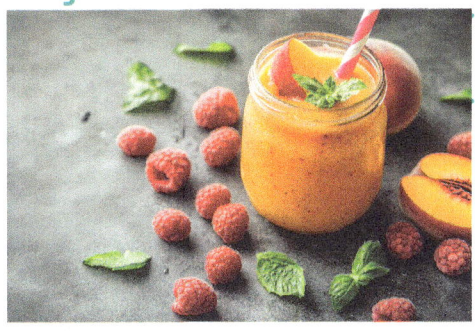

Instructions:

1. Wash the raspberries and peaches if using fresh. Measure out the frozen fruits if using frozen.
2. In a blender, combine the peaches, raspberries, lactose-free yogurt, lactose-free milk (or almond milk), and honey or maple syrup. Add ice cubes if a thicker texture is desired. Blend on high speed until smooth and creamy, about 30 seconds to 1 minute.
3. Pour the smoothie into a glass and serve immediately.
4. Optionally, garnish with a few extra raspberries or a slice of peach.

Coconut Blueberry Smoothie

Serves: 1 | **Prep:** 5 minutes
Cook: No cooking required

Nutrition:

Cal 220| **Fat** 12g
Carb 25g | **Protein** 7g

Ingredients:

- ½ cup blueberries (fresh or frozen)
- ½ cup coconut milk (from a carton)
- ½ cup lactose-free yogurt
- 1 tsp chia seeds (optional, for added fiber)
- 1 tsp maple syrup (optional, for sweetness)
- ¼ cup ice cubes (optional)

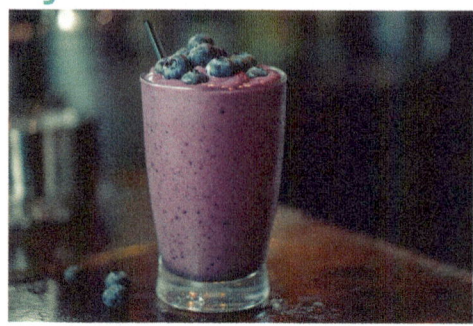

Instructions:

1. In a blender, combine the blueberries, coconut milk, lactose-free yogurt, chia seeds (if using), maple syrup (if using), and ice cubes.
2. Blend on high speed for about 30 seconds to 1 minute, or until smooth and creamy.
3. Pour the smoothie into a glass and serve immediately.
4. Optionally, garnish with a few extra blueberries or a sprinkle of chia seeds.

Chapter 1: Breakfasts

Coconut Lime Smoothie

Serves: 1 | **Prep:** 5 minutes
Cook: No cooking required

Nutrition:

Cal 180 | **Fat** 10g
Carb 25g | **Protein** 6g

Ingredients:

- ½cup coconut milk (from a carton)
- ½cup lactose-free yogurt
- 1tbsp fresh lime juice
- 1tsp lime zest (optional, for more tang)
- 1tsp maple syrup (optional, for sweetness)
- ¼cup ice cubes (optional, for a thicker texture)
- Fresh mint leaves (optional, for garnish)

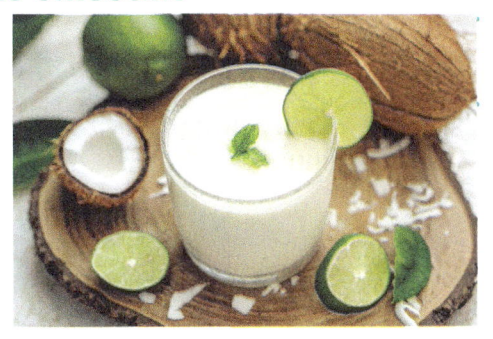

Instructions:

1. In a blender, combine the coconut milk, lactose-free yogurt, lime juice, lime zest (if using), maple syrup (if using), and ice cubes.
2. Blend on high speed for about 30 seconds to 1 minute until smooth and creamy.
3. Pour the smoothie into a glass and serve immediately.
4. Optionally, garnish with fresh mint leaves or an extra sprinkle of lime zest.

Chapter 2: Snacks
Pumpkin Spice Protein Balls

Serves: 12
Prep: 10 minutes | **Chill Time:** 1 hou

Nutrition:

Cal 120 | **Fat** 9g
Carb 10g | **Protein** 8g

Ingredients:

- ½cup almond butter
- ¼cup pumpkin puree (ensure it's pure, no additives)
- ¼cup gluten-free oats
- ¼cup unsweetened shredded coconut
- ¼cup raw pumpkin seeds
- 2tbsp chopped walnuts or pecans
- 2tbsp chia seeds (optional, for added texture and fiber)
- 1 scoop vanilla protein powder (check for FODMAP-friendly brands)
- 2tbsp maple syrup (or to taste)
- 1tsp pumpkin spice (cinnamon, nutmeg, ginger, and cloves)
- A pinch of salt
- 1-2tbsp water (if needed to adjust consistency)

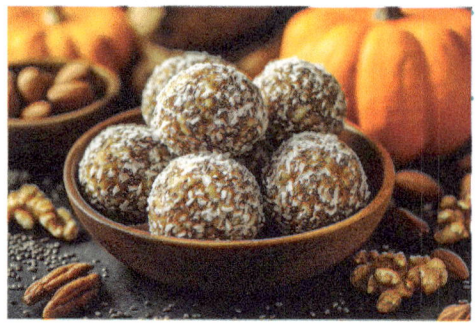

Instructions:

1. In a large mixing bowl, combine the almond butter, pumpkin puree, gluten-free oats, unsweetened shredded coconut, pumpkin seeds, walnuts (or pecans), chia seeds (if using), protein powder, pumpkin spice, and salt.
2. Stir well until all the ingredients are combined. If the mixture feels too dry, add 1-2tbsp of water to adjust the consistency.
3. Using your hands or a small spoon, scoop out portions of the mixture and roll them into 1-inch balls.
4. Place the protein balls on a plate or baking sheet lined with parchment paper and refrigerate for at least 30 minutes to firm up.
5. Once chilled, enjoy it as a quick snack or post-workout energy bite! Store any leftovers in an airtight container in the fridge for up to a week.

Chapter 2: Snacks

Salted Caramel Peanut Candy Bars

Serves: 15
Prep: 15 minutes | **Cook:** 20 minute

Nutrition:

Cal 180 | **Fat** 14g
Carb 18g | **Protein** 5g

Ingredients:

For the Base:
- 1cup gluten-free all-purpose flour
- ¼cup lactose-free butter, softened
- 2tbsp granulated sugar
- ¼tsp salt

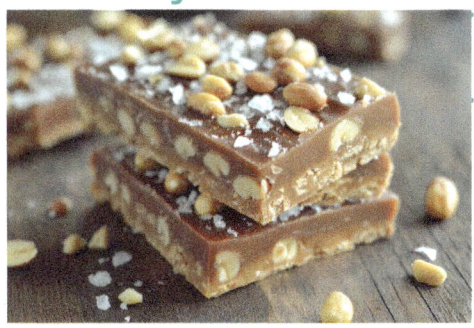

For the Salted Caramel Layer:
- ½cup lactose-free butter
- ½cup brown sugar, packed
- ¼cup pure maple syrup
- ¼cup lactose-free heavy cream
- ½tsp sea salt
- 1cup roasted, unsalted peanuts

Instructions:

1. Preheat the oven to 350°F (180°C). Grease an 8x8-inch baking pan and line it with parchment paper.
2. In a medium bowl, combine the gluten-free flour, softened lactose-free butter, sugar, and salt. Mix until the dough forms.
3. Press the dough evenly into the prepared baking pan to create the base.
4. Bake for 10-12 minutes or until the edges are golden. Set aside to cool.
5. In a medium saucepan, melt the butter over medium heat. Add the brown sugar, maple syrup, and lactose-free heavy cream. Stir until the mixture is smooth.
6. Let the mixture come to a boil, and cook for 4-5 minutes, stirring occasionally, until the caramel thickens.
7. Remove from heat, stir in the sea salt, and fold in the roasted peanuts.
8. Pour the caramel-peanut mixture over the cooled base, spreading it evenly. Let it cool for 15-20 minutes.
9. Refrigerate the candy bars for at least 2 hours, or until the layers are fully set.
10. Once chilled, remove from the pan and cut into 16 bars.

Muesli Bars

Serves: 15
Prep: 25 minutes | **Cook:** 15 minute

Nutrition:

Cal 188 | **Fat** 15g
Carb 10g | **Protein** 4g

Ingredients:

- 1cup rolled oats
- ½cup sunflower seeds
- ½cup pumpkin seeds
- ½cup sesame seeds
- 1tbsp flax seeds
- 1cup desiccated coconut
- 1tsp ground cinnamon
- Olive oil spread
- ½cup rice malt syrup

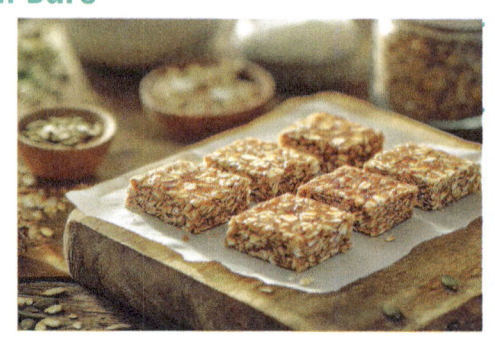

Instructions:

1. In a small saucepan, melt and combine olive oil spread, rice malt syrup, and cinnamon.
2. In a large non-stick fry pan, combine oats, seeds, and coconut and toast over a low heat for approximately 5-10 minutes.
3. Add dry mix to the oil-syrup-cinnamon mix and mix until combined.
4. Press into a slice tin lined with baking paper and freeze for approximately 20 minutes until set.
5. Cut into squares. You can cut the baking paper, lining the tin, into strips, and wrap the bars individually.
6. Store in the freezer until use.

Note:

- If your child doesn't like 'bits' in their baked goods, use a food processor to combine and break down the mixture.
- Use this recipe as a base and experiment with adding other low-FODMAP ingredients, such as dried cranberries or nuts.

Savory Muffin

Serves: 12
Prep: 10 minutes | **Cook:** 20 minute

Nutrition:

Cal 264 | **Fat** 11g
Carb 36g | **Protein** 6g

Ingredients:

- 1¼cup tapioca flour
- 1¼cup maize flour
- 5¼tsp baking powder
- 1¾ tsp xanthan gum
- ¾ cup oat bran
- 3 eggs
- ¾cup cream
- ¾cup milk, low-fat, lactose-free milk
- 1cup feta cheese, crumbled
- 1cup capsicum, red, finely diced
- ¾cup basil leaves (roughly chopped)
- Grated cheese to top each muffin
- Paprika to top each muffin

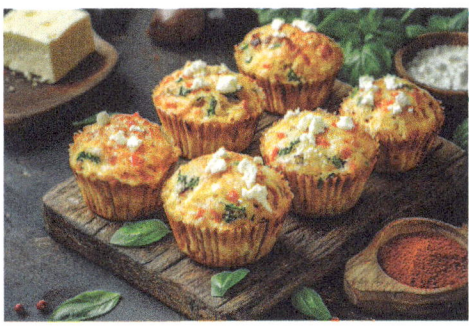

Instructions:

1. Preheat oven to 160°C/320°F and on a lower shelf of the oven, half-fill a baking tray with boiling water (see tip below).
2. Sift flour, baking powder, and xanthan gum into a large bowl, then add the bran (mix again).
3. In a separate bowl, whisk eggs with the cream and milk.
4. Add capsicum, crumbled feta, and basil to the egg mixture.
5. Make a well in the flour mix and fold wet mix into the dry ingredients (you may have to add more milk to achieve dough that is slightly sloppy but not too wet).
6. Place large muffin cases in a muffin tray and spray well with canola oil.
7. Fill muffin cases (see tip below) and tap down the top surface with a wet finger.
8. Sprinkle the top of each muffin with grated cheese, then paprika.
9. Bake for about 17 minutes until golden brown (an inserted skewer should be clean when removed).
10. Cool in the tray for 5 minutes, then place on a wire rack to cool further.

Peanut Butter Energy Bars

Serves: 12 | **Prep:** 70 minutes
Cook: No cooking required

Nutrition:

Cal 217 | **Fat** 12g
Carb 20g | **Protein** 6g

Ingredients:

- ½cup natural peanut butter (no added sugar or salt)
- ½cup maple syrup
- 1cup rolled oats, lightly toasted
- ½cup puffed brown rice
- ½cup quinoa flakes
- ½cup almonds, lightly toasted, chopped
- ¼cup dried cranberries, chopped
- ¼cup dried banana, chopped
- 1tbsp coconut flakes, lightly toasted
- 1tbsp chia seeds
- 1tbsp sunflower seeds

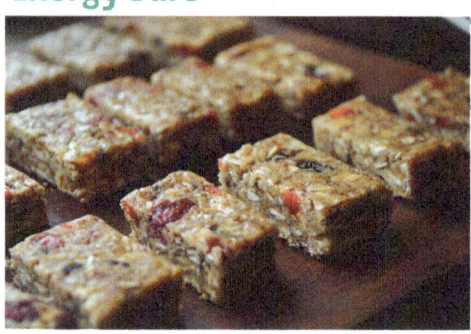

Instructions:

1. Spray an 8x8-inch slice tray with cooking spray and line with baking paper, set aside.
2. In a small saucepan, heat peanut butter and maple syrup over low heat, stirring until well combined.
3. In a large bowl, combine dry ingredients. Pour peanut and maple syrup mixture over dry ingredients and stir until well combined.
4. Transfer mixture into prepared tray, pressing down with slightly wet hands to ensure mixture is flat and tightly packed together.
5. Refrigerate for at least 1 hour before gently removing from the tray and slicing into bars.

Note:

- Store bars in an airtight container in the fridge.
- To make bars nut-free, replace peanut butter with sunflower seed butter and omit almonds.
- To make bars gluten-free, substitute rolled oats for quinoa or millet flakes.

Chapter 2: Snacks

Mixed Berry & Yogurt Granola Bar

Serves: 12
Prep: 5 minutes | **Cook:** 30 minutes

Nutrition:

Cal 179 | **Fat** 10g
Carb 19g | **Protein** 4g

Ingredients:

- 2cups rolled oats
- ¼cup finely shredded coconut
- 2½tbsp macadamia nut meal
- 2½tbsp chia seeds
- 1 egg white
- 2½tbsp peanut oil
- ¼cup pure maple syrup
- 5oz mixed berries
- 7oz plain Greek/natural yogurt
- 1.75oz white chocolate melts, melted

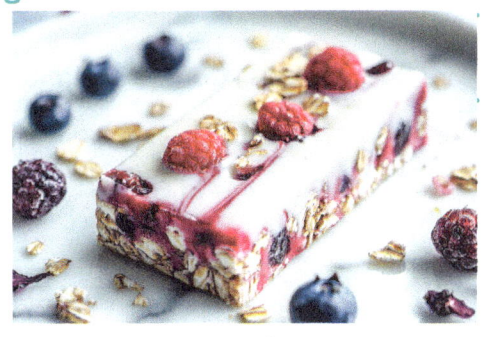

Instructions:

1. Preheat oven to 180°C/356°F. Line a 6x10-inch slice pan with baking paper.
2. Combine all ingredients in a large mixing bowl.
3. Press mixture into pan.
4. Bake for 30 minutes or until golden.
5. Drizzle with melted white chocolate and cut into slices to serve.

Spiced Molasses Cookies

Serves: 30
Prep: 75 minutes | **Cook:** 10 minute

Nutrition:

Cal 114 | **Fat** 5g
Carb 17g | **Protein** 0g

Ingredients:

- ¾ cup butter or margarine, melted
- 1tsp stevia
- 1 egg
- ¼ cup molasses
- 2 cups gluten-free plain flour
- 2tsp baking powder
- ½ tsp salt
- 1tsp ground cinnamon
- ½ tsp ground nutmeg
- ½ tsp ground ginger

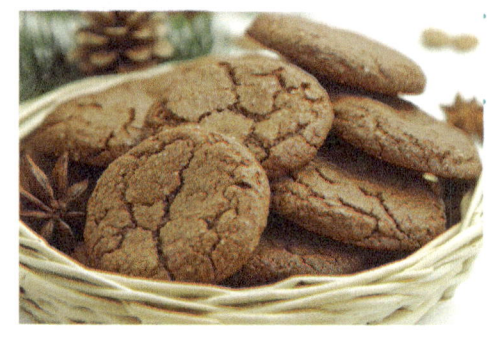

Instructions:

1. In a large bowl, combine melted butter, sugar, and egg and mix until smooth. Stir in molasses, flour, baking powder, salt, cinnamon, and allspice and stir until mixture combines into dough. Cover dough with plastic wrap and refrigerate for at least 1 hour, or until dough is firm.
2. Meanwhile, preheat oven to 180°C/356°F and line a large baking tray with baking paper.
3. Divide dough into 30 walnut-sized pieces and roll into balls. Place dough balls on the baking tray ~2 inch apart. Do not flatten dough: cookies will spread out as they bake.
4. Bake cookies in oven for ~10 minutes or until tops of cookies begin to crack. Leave cookies on tray to cool slightly before transferring onto a wire cooling rack.

Peanut Butter and Hemp Seed Protein Balls

Serves: 12 | **Prep:** 10 minutes
Cook: No cooking required

Nutrition:

Cal 286 | **Fat** 10g
Carb 6g | **Protein** 5g

Ingredients:

- ½ cup natural peanut butter (no added salt or sugar)
- 2 tbsp pure maple syrup or sorghum syrup
- 1 tsp vanilla extract
- ⅓ cup hulled hemp seeds
- 1⅓ tbsp oat bran
- 2 tbsp linseeds (flax seeds)
- 3 squares dark chocolate, chopped into small chunks

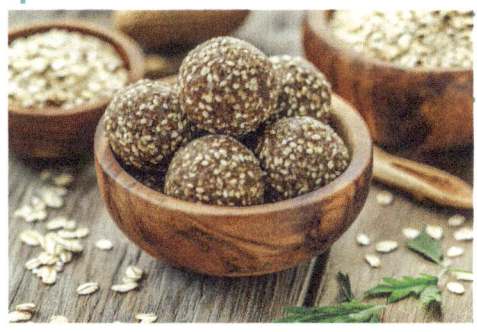

Instructions:

1. In a mixing bowl or food processor, thoroughly combine all the ingredients. The mixture should hold together when squeezed into a ball.
2. Press into 1-inch balls and roll in your hands until well formed.
3. Store in the fridge in a sealed container for up to 2 weeks, or wrap individually and freeze for up to 3 months.

Note:

- Try substituting walnuts for peanut butter by making your own walnut butter in a food processor. You'll add more diversity to your diet and your gut will love it.
- For a nut-free version, finely blitz lightly roasted pumpkin seeds (pepitas) and add 1–1½ tbsp melted coconut oil.
- Double the batch and store them in the freezer.

Cranberry Orange Protein Balls

Serves: 12 | **Prep:** 10 minutes
Chill Time: 2 hours

Nutrition:

Cal 137 | **Fat** 10g
Carb 10g | **Protein** 3g

Ingredients:

- ½ cup raw almonds
- ½ cup raw walnuts
- ¼ cup unsweetened flaked coconut
- 1.5 to 2.5 large-pitted dates
- ½ cup juice-sweetened dried cranberries
- 1 tsp orange zest
- ¼ cup sunflower seed butter or almond butter
- 1½ tbsp coconut oil or flax oil
- 1 scoop hemp protein powder or protein powder of choice
- 1 tsp pure vanilla extract
- A pinch of salt

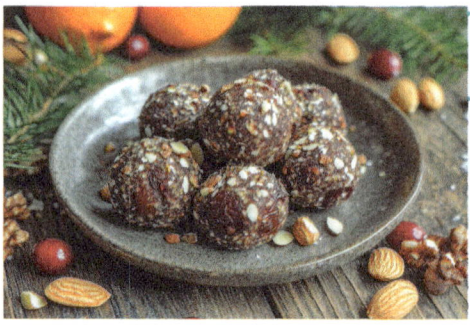

Instructions

1. Add all ingredients into your food processor and process until a thick dough-like mixture forms.
2. Transfer the ball mixture to a sealable container and refrigerate for at least 2 hours. This helps the ingredients set up so that it's easier to form the balls. If you try to form the balls right away, they will often crumble and not hold together.
3. Store the balls in a sealable bag or container in the refrigerator or freezer.

Chapter 2: Snacks

Fig and Date Energy Balls

Serves: 12 | **Prep:** 10 minutes
Chill Time: 2 hours

Nutrition:

Cal 122 | **Fat** 8g
Carb 12g | **Protein** 3g

Ingredients:

- ½ cup Medjool dates pitted
- ½ cup dried figs
- 1¼ cups of raw cashews
- ½ cup unsweetened shredded coconut
- ½ tbsp chia seeds
- ½ tbsp hemp seeds
- 1 tsp pure vanilla extract
- A pinch of sea salt

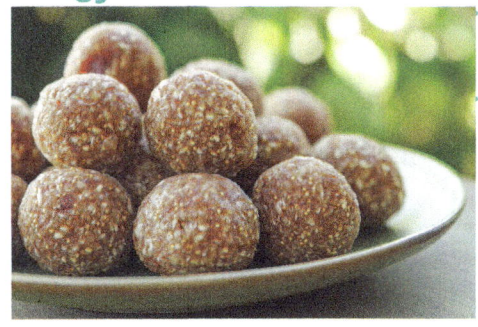

Instructions:

1. Add all ingredients for the fig and date balls to a food processor. Process until a sticky dough forms. If needed, stop the food processor to scrape the sides to help it thoroughly process the mixture.
2. If the mixture is very sticky, refrigerate it for 2 hours before rolling the dough into balls.
3. Roll dough into desired-sized balls, and enjoy!
4. Balls should be stored in a sealable bag or container in the refrigerator or freezer.

Chapter 3: Lunch
Quinoa Tabbouleh

Serves: 2
Prep: 15 minutes | **Cook:** 15 minutes

Nutrition:

Cal 280 | **Fat** 16g
Carb 32g | **Protein** 6g

Ingredients:

- ½ cup quinoa, rinsed
- 1 cup water
- ½ cucumber, diced
- 1 cup cherry tomatoes, halved
- ¼ cup fresh parsley, finely chopped
- 2 tbsp fresh mint, finely chopped
- 2 tbsp lemon juice (freshly squeezed)
- 2 tbsp extra-virgin olive oil
- Salt and pepper to taste

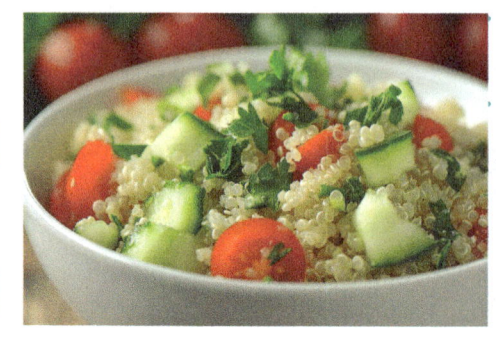

Instructions:

1. In a medium saucepan, combine the rinsed quinoa and water. Bring to a boil over medium-high heat. Once boiling, reduce the heat to low, cover the saucepan, and let the quinoa simmer for about 12-15 minutes, or until all the water is absorbed and the quinoa is tender. Once cooked, remove the saucepan from the heat and let the quinoa sit covered for 5 minutes. Then, fluff the quinoa with a fork and let it cool to room temperature.
2. While the quinoa is cooling, dice the cucumber and halve the cherry tomatoes. Finely chop the parsley and mint leaves.
3. In a small bowl, whisk together the freshly squeezed lemon juice, extra-virgin olive oil, salt, and pepper until well combined.
4. In a large mixing bowl, combine the cooled quinoa, diced cucumber, halved cherry tomatoes, chopped parsley, and mint. Pour the dressing over the quinoa and vegetables, and toss gently to combine all the ingredients evenly.
5. Taste the tabbouleh and adjust the seasoning with additional salt, pepper, or lemon juice if needed. Serve immediately or refrigerate for up to 1 hour before serving to allow the flavors to meld together.

Grilled Lamb Chops with Mint

Serves: 2 | **Prep:** 45 minutes to 2 hours (optional) | **Cook:** 20 minutes

Nutrition:

Cal 450 | **Fat** 35g
Carb 4g | **Protein** 30g

Ingredients:

- 4 lamb chops
- 2tbsp fresh mint, finely chopped
- 2tbsp fresh parsley, finely chopped
- 1tbsp garlic-infused olive oil
- 2tbsp olive oil
- 1tbsp lemon juice (freshly squeezed)
- Salt and pepper to taste
- Lemon wedges for serving (optional)

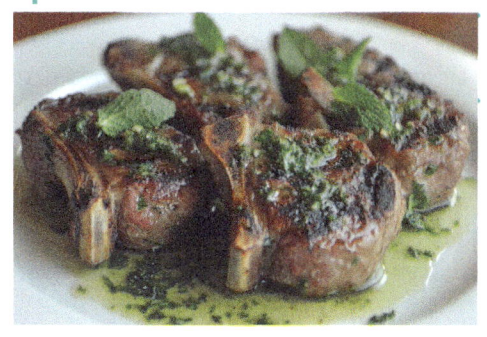

Instructions:

1. In a small bowl, combine the chopped mint, parsley, garlic-infused oil, olive oil, lemon juice, salt, and pepper. Mix well.
2. Marinate the lamb chops (optional). Place the lamb chops in a shallow dish or a resealable plastic bag. Pour the marinade over the lamb chops, ensuring they are evenly coated. Cover the dish and let the lamb chops marinate in the refrigerator for at least 30 minutes, up to 2 hours for a more intense flavor.
3. Preheat your grill to medium-high heat (around 375°F to 400°F). If using a grill pan, preheat it over medium-high heat on the stovetop.
4. Remove the lamb chops from the marinade and shake off any excess. Place the lamb chops on the grill or grill pan. Grill for about 4-5 minutes per side, depending on the thickness of the chops and your desired level of doneness. For medium-rare, aim for an internal temperature of 135°F (57°C); for medium, aim for 145°F (63°C).
5. Once cooked to your desired doneness, remove the lamb chops from the grill and let them rest for 5 minutes. This allows the juices to redistribute throughout the meat, ensuring a tender and flavorful result.
6. Pair the lamb chops with your favorite sides, such as roasted vegetables.

Notes:

- The nutritional value of the dish is calculated without the side dish.

Shrimp Saganaki

Serves: 2
Prep: 10 minutes | **Cook:** 15 minutes

Nutrition:

Cal 300 | **Fat** 15g
Carb 8g | **Protein** 28g

Ingredients:

- 12 large shrimp, peeled and deveined
- 1 tbsp garlic-infused olive oil
- 1 can (14.5oz) diced tomatoes (choose a brand without onion or garlic)
- ¼ cup crumbled feta cheese (lactose-free if needed)
- ¼ cup white wine (optional)
- 1 tsp dried oregano
- 1 tsp dried thyme
- ¼ tsp red pepper flakes (optional)
- Salt and pepper to taste
- Fresh parsley, chopped for garnish
- Lemon wedges for serving

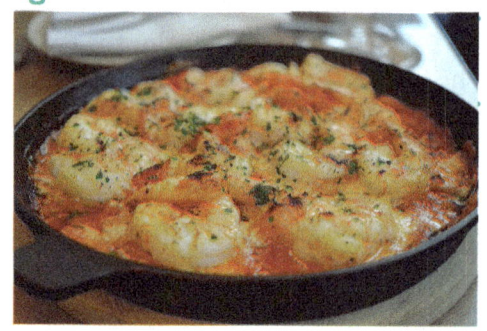

Instructions:

1. Rinse the shrimp under cold water and pat them dry with a paper towel. Set aside.
2. Heat the garlic-infused olive oil in a large skillet over medium heat. Add the canned diced tomatoes (including the juice), dried oregano, dried thyme, and red pepper flakes (if using). If you're using white wine, add it at this stage. Stir the mixture and let it simmer for 5-7 minutes, allowing the flavors to meld together. Cook until the sauce slightly thickens.
3. Add the prepared shrimp to the skillet, arranging them in a single layer over the tomato sauce.
   Cook the shrimp for 2-3 minutes on one side, then flip them and cook for an additional 2-3 minutes, or until they are pink and opaque.
4. Sprinkle the crumbled feta cheese over the shrimp and tomato mixture. Reduce the heat to low, cover the skillet, and cook for an additional 2 minutes until the feta is slightly melted and the shrimp are fully cooked.
5. Remove the skillet from the heat. Garnish with fresh chopped parsley and serve with lemon wedges on the side.

Mediterranean Chicken Skewers

Serves: 2 | **Prep:** 45 minutes to 2 hours (optional) | **Cook:** 15 minutes

Nutrition:

Cal 400 | **Fat** 24g
Carb 10g | **Protein** 40g

Ingredients:

- 2 boneless, skinless chicken breasts, cut into 1-inch cubes
- 1 red bell pepper, cut into 1-inch pieces
- 1 zucchini, sliced into rounds
- 1 small red onion, cut into 1-inch pieces (use only the green tops for low-FODMAP, or omit)
- ¼ cup olive oil
- 2 tbsp lemon juice (freshly squeezed)
- 1 tbsp red wine vinegar
- 1 tbsp garlic-infused olive oil
- 1 tsp dried oregano
- 1 tsp dried thyme
- Salt and pepper to taste
- Wooden or metal skewers

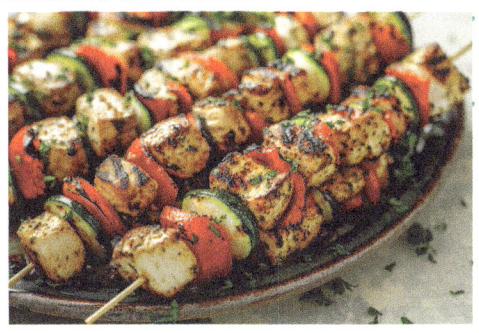

Instructions:

1. Prepare the Marinade. In a medium bowl, whisk together the olive oil, lemon juice, red wine vinegar, garlic-infused olive oil, dried oregano, dried thyme, salt, and pepper.
2. Add the chicken cubes to the bowl with the marinade, making sure all pieces are well coated.
Cover the bowl with plastic wrap and let the chicken marinate rest in the refrigerator for at least 30 minutes, up to 2 hours for the best flavor. If you're short on time, you can proceed immediately to the next step but marinating enhances the flavor.
3. Prepare the Skewers. If using wooden skewers, soak them in water for 15-20 minutes to prevent them from burning on the grill. Thread the marinated chicken cubes, red bell pepper pieces, zucchini slices, and onion pieces (if using) onto the skewers, alternating the ingredients as you go.
4. Preheat your grill to medium-high heat (around 375°F to 400°F). If using a grill pan, preheat it over medium-high heat on the stovetop.
5. Place the skewers on the preheated grill. Cook for about 4-5 minutes on each side, turning occasionally, until the chicken is fully cooked and

has nice grill marks. The internal temperature of the chicken should reach 165°F (74°C).
6. Once the chicken is cooked through, remove the skewers from the grill.
7. Serve the Mediterranean chicken skewers with a side of quinoa, rice, or a simple salad. Garnish with extra lemon wedges if desired.

Notes:

- The nutritional value of the dish is calculated without the side dish.

Salmon with Dill and Lemon

Serves: 2
Prep: 10 minutes | **Cook:** 20 minute

Nutrition:

Cal 400 | **Fat** 24g
Carb 4g | **Protein** 36g

Ingredients:

- 2 salmon fillets (about 6oz each)
- 2tbsp fresh dill, chopped
- 1 lemon (zested and juiced)
- 1tbsp olive oil
- Salt and pepper to taste
- Lemon wedges for serving

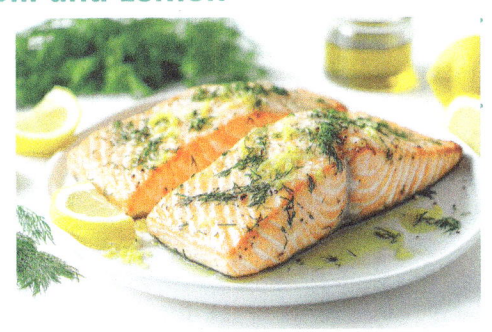

Instructions:

1. Preheat your oven to 375°F (190°C).
2. Lightly grease a baking dish with olive oil or line it with parchment paper. This will help prevent the salmon from sticking and make for easier cleanup.
3. Place the salmon fillets in the prepared baking dish, skin-side down. Drizzle the fillets with olive oil, ensuring they are evenly coated. Sprinkle the chopped fresh dill over the salmon fillets. Zest the lemon over the fillets, then squeeze the lemon juice evenly over the top. Season with salt and pepper to taste.
4. Bake the Salmon. Place the baking dish in the preheated oven. Bake the salmon for 15-20 minutes, or until the salmon is opaque and flakes easily with a fork. The exact cooking time may vary depending on the thickness of the fillets.
5. Once cooked, remove the salmon from the oven. Serve the salmon fillets hot with extra lemon wedges on the side for added flavor.
6. Pair with your favorite low-FODMAP side dishes, such as roasted vegetables, steamed asparagus, or a simple quinoa salad.

Notes:

- The nutritional value of the dish is calculated without the side dish.

Chicken Piccata

Serves: 2
Prep: 10 minutes | **Cook:** 20 minute

Nutrition:

Cal 450 | **Fat** 30g
Carb 12g | **Protein** 35g

Ingredients:

- 2 boneless, skinless chicken breasts, pounded to ½-inch thickness
- ¼ cup gluten-free flour
- 2 tbsp olive oil
- ½ cup chicken broth (low-sodium)
- ¼ cup lemon juice (freshly squeezed)
- ¼ cup dry white wine (optional)
- 2 tbsp capers, drained
- 2 tbsp unsalted butter (or lactose-free butter if needed)
- Salt and pepper to taste
- Fresh parsley, chopped for garnish
- Lemon slices for garnish (optional)

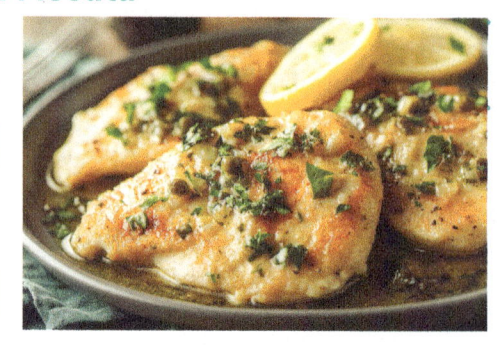

Instructions:

1. Season the chicken breasts with salt and pepper on both sides. Dredge the chicken in the gluten-free flour, ensuring it is evenly coated. Shake off any excess flour.
2. Heat the olive oil in a large skillet over medium-high heat. Add the chicken breasts to the skillet and cook for about 4-5 minutes on each side, or until they are golden brown and cooked through. The internal temperature should reach 165°F (74°C). Once cooked, transfer the chicken to a plate and cover with foil to keep warm.
3. Make the sauce. In the same skillet, reduce the heat to medium. Add the chicken broth, lemon juice, and white wine (if using). Stir to combine and scrape up any browned bits from the bottom of the pan. Let the mixture simmer for about 2-3 minutes, allowing the sauce to reduce slightly.
4. Stir in the capers and unsalted butter. Continue to simmer for another 2-3 minutes, until the sauce thickens slightly and becomes glossy.
5. Return the cooked chicken breasts to the skillet, spooning the sauce over them to coat. Allow the chicken to warm through for another minute or two.

Chapter 3: Lunch

6. Transfer the chicken to serving plates, spooning the sauce over the top. Garnish with fresh parsley and lemon slices if desired.
7. Serve the Chicken Piccata with a side of gluten-free pasta, steamed vegetables, or a light salad.

Notes:

- The nutritional value of the dish is calculated without the side dish.

Greek-Style Meatballs

Serves: 4
Prep: 20 minutes | **Cook:** 25 minute

Nutrition:

Cal 400 | **Fat** 28g
Carb 10g | **Protein** 30g

Ingredients:

For the Meatballs:
- 1lb ground beef or lamb (or a mix of both)
- ¼cup gluten-free breadcrumbs (ensure they are low-FODMAP)
- ¼cup lactose-free feta cheese, crumbled (optional)
- 1 large egg
- 2tbsp fresh parsley, chopped
- 1tbsp fresh mint, chopped
- 1tsp dried oregano
- 1tbsp garlic-infused olive oil (for low-FODMAP)
- Salt and pepper to taste

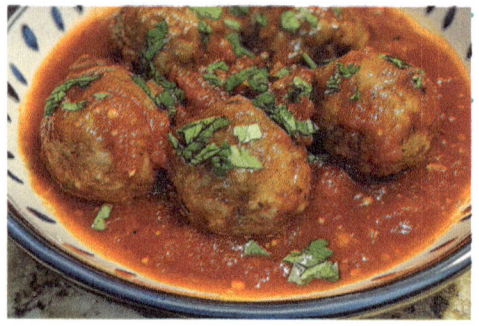

For the Tomato Sauce:
- 1can (14.5oz) diced tomatoes (choose a brand without onion or garlic)
- 1tbsp tomato paste (ensure it's low-FODMAP)
- 1tbsp garlic-infused olive oil
- 1tsp dried oregano
- 1tsp dried basil
- Salt and pepper to taste

Instructions:

1. Prepare the meatball mixture. In a large mixing bowl, combine the ground beef or lamb, gluten-free breadcrumbs, crumbled feta cheese (if using), egg, chopped parsley, chopped mint, dried oregano, salt, and pepper. Add 1 tablespoon of garlic-infused olive oil to the mixture. Use your hands or a spoon to thoroughly mix all the ingredients together until well combined.
2. Form the meatballs. Preheat your oven to 375°F (190°C). Line a baking sheet with parchment paper or lightly grease it with olive oil. Form the meat mixture into small meatballs, about 1 to 1.5 inches in diameter. You should get about 16-20 meatballs, depending on size. Place the meatballs on the prepared baking sheet, ensuring they are evenly spaced.
3. Place the baking sheet with the meatballs in the preheated oven. Bake for 20-25 minutes, or until the meatballs are browned on the outside

and cooked through. The internal temperature should reach 160°F (71°C).
4. Prepare the tomato sauce. While the meatballs are baking, heat 1 tablespoon of garlic-infused olive oil in a medium-sized saucepan over medium heat. Add the diced tomatoes (with their juice), tomato paste, dried oregano, dried basil, salt, and pepper. Stir to combine all the ingredients, then bring the mixture to a simmer. Reduce the heat to low and let the sauce simmer for about 10-15 minutes, stirring occasionally, until it thickens slightly.
5. Once the meatballs are fully cooked, remove them from the oven. Carefully transfer the meatballs to the saucepan with the tomato sauce. Gently stir to coat the meatballs with the sauce, then let them simmer together for an additional 5 minutes to absorb the flavors.
6. Serve the Greek-style meatballs hot, garnished with extra chopped parsley if desired.
7. These meatballs pair beautifully with gluten-free pasta or rice.

Notes:

- The nutritional value of the dish is calculated without the side dish.

Chicken and Gnocchi Casserole

Serves: 2
Prep: 15 minutes | **Cook:** 30 minute

Nutrition:

Cal 500 | **Fat** 25g
Carb 50g | Protein 30g

Ingredients:

- 1 package (about 10oz) gluten-free gnocchi
- 1 boneless, skinless chicken breast (about 6oz), diced into bite-sized pieces
- 1 tbsp garlic-infused olive oil
- ½ cup lactose-free milk
- ½ cup low-FODMAP chicken broth
- ½ cup lactose-free cheddar cheese, shredded
- ½ cup fresh spinach, chopped
- ¼ cup green tops of scallions, chopped
- 1 tbsp gluten-free flour
- 1 tbsp unsalted butter (or lactose-free butter)
- Salt and pepper to taste
- ¼ tsp dried thyme (optional)
- ¼ tsp dried oregano (optional)

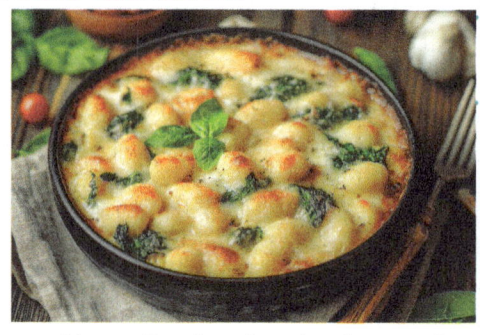

Instructions:

1. Preheat your oven to 375°F (190°C).
2. Bring a large pot of salted water to a boil. Add the gluten-free gnocchi and cook according to the package instructions, usually until they float to the surface (about 2-3 minutes). Drain the gnocchi and set aside.
3. In a large skillet, heat the garlic-infused olive oil over medium heat. Add the diced chicken breast and cook until browned and cooked through, about 5-7 minutes. Remove the chicken from the skillet and set aside.
4. In the same skillet, melt the butter over medium heat. Stir in the gluten-free flour and cook for 1-2 minutes to create a roux. Gradually whisk in the low-FODMAP chicken broth and lactose-free milk, stirring constantly until the sauce thickens. Add the shredded lactose-free cheddar cheese, stirring until melted and smooth. Season the sauce with salt, pepper, thyme, and oregano to taste.
5. In a large mixing bowl, combine the cooked gnocchi, cooked chicken, chopped spinach, and green tops of scallions. Pour the cheese sauce over the mixture and stir until everything is well coated.

6. Transfer the mixture to a greased baking dish. Bake in the preheated oven for 15-20 minutes, or until the casserole is bubbly and golden on top.
7. Remove the casserole from the oven and let it cool for a few minutes before serving.

Warm Chicken and Roast Vegetable Salad

Serves: 2
Prep: 15 minutes | **Cook:** 30 minute

Nutrition:

Cal 400 | **Fat** 25g
Carb 15g | **Protein** 35g

Ingredients:

- 2 boneless, skinless chicken breasts (about 6oz each)
- 1 medium zucchini, sliced into rounds
- 1 red bell pepper, sliced into strips
- 1 small eggplant, cubed
- 1cup cherry tomatoes, halved
- 1tbsp garlic-infused olive oil
- 2cups mixed greens (such as spinach, arugula, or lettuce)
- ¼cup crumbled lactose-free feta cheese (optional)
- Salt and pepper to taste
- 2tbsp extra virgin olive oil
- 1tbsp lemon juice (freshly squeezed)
- 1tsp Dijon mustard (check for low-FODMAP ingredients)
- 1tsp maple syrup (optional for sweetness)
- Salt and pepper to taste

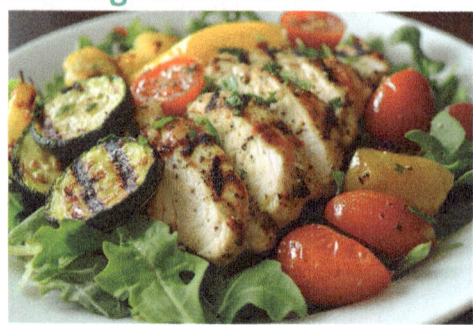

Instructions:

1. Preheat your oven to 400°F (200°C).
2. Place the zucchini slices, red bell pepper strips, eggplant cubes, and halved cherry tomatoes on a baking sheet. Drizzle the vegetables with the garlic-infused olive oil, and season with salt and pepper. Toss to coat the vegetables evenly. Roast the vegetables in the preheated oven for 20-25 minutes, or until they are tender and slightly caramelized. Stir the vegetables halfway through cooking to ensure even roasting.
3. While the vegetables are roasting, heat a grill pan or skillet over medium-high heat. Season the chicken breasts with salt and pepper. Grill the chicken for about 5-7 minutes per side, or until fully cooked and the internal temperature reaches 165°F (74°C). Once cooked, remove the chicken from the heat and let it rest for a few minutes before slicing it into thin strips.
4. In a small bowl, whisk together the extra virgin olive oil, lemon juice, Dijon mustard, and maple syrup (if using). Season the dressing with salt and pepper to taste.

5. Divide the mixed greens between two plates or large salad bowls. Top each salad with roasted vegetables and sliced chicken. Drizzle the dressing over the salad, and sprinkle with crumbled lactose-free feta cheese if using.
6. Serve the warm chicken and roast vegetable salad immediately.

Asian-Inspired Quinoa Salad

Serves: 2
Prep: 15 minutes | **Cook:** 15 minutes

Nutrition:

Cal 350 | **Fat** 20g
Carb 55g | **Protein** 10g

Ingredients:

- ½cup quinoa, rinsed
- 1cup water
- ½ red bell pepper, thinly sliced
- ½ cucumber, thinly sliced
- 1 small carrot, julienned
- ¼cup green tops of scallions, chopped
- 1tbsp sesame seeds, toasted
- ½cup firm tofu or cooked chicken breast, diced (optional for added protein)
- 2tbsp garlic-infused olive oil
- 1tbsp soy sauce (ensure it's gluten-free and low-FODMAP)
- 1tbsp rice vinegar
- 1tsp sesame oil
- 1tsp maple syrup or sugar
- ½tsp fresh ginger, grated (optional)
- Salt and pepper to taste

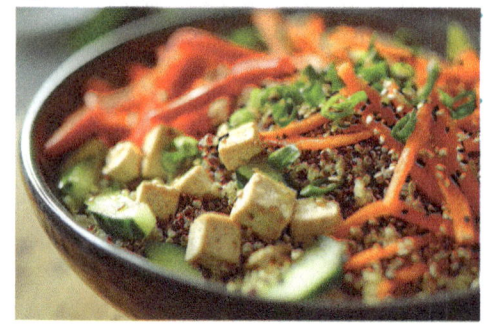

Instructions:

1. In a medium saucepan, combine the rinsed quinoa and water. Bring to a boil over medium-high heat. Once boiling, reduce the heat to low, cover, and simmer for about 15 minutes, or until the quinoa has absorbed all the water and is tender. Remove from heat, fluff with a fork, and let it cool to room temperature.
2. While the quinoa is cooking, prepare the vegetables by slicing the red bell pepper, cucumber, and carrot. Chop the green tops of the scallions.
3. In a small bowl, whisk together the garlic-infused olive oil, soy sauce, rice vinegar, sesame oil, maple syrup, and grated ginger (if using). Season with salt and pepper to taste.
4. In a large bowl, combine the cooked quinoa, sliced vegetables, and tofu or chicken (if using). Pour the dressing over the salad and toss to combine. Sprinkle the toasted sesame seeds on top.
5. Serve the salad immediately or chill it in the refrigerator for a bit to allow the flavors to meld.

Tandoori Chicken

Serves: 2
Prep: 25 minutes | **Cook:** 30 minute

Nutrition:

Cal 616 | **Fat** 39g
Carb 29g | **Protein** 14g

Ingredients

- 2oz plain Greek yogurt (or lactose-free yogurt if you malabsorb lactose)
- 1tsp tomato paste
- ½tsp paprika
- ½tsp ground coriander
- ½tsp salt
- 10.5oz chicken breast, in thick slices
- 1tbsp olive oil
- 1lb Kent/Japanese pumpkin, cut into thick slices
- 1/5cup fresh lime juice
- 1tbsp ginger, peeled and finely chopped
- 1cup of coriander leaves
- Steamed rice, to serve

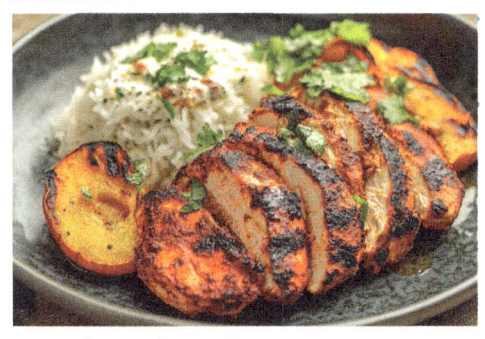

Instructions:

1. Preheat the oven to 230°C/450°F.
2. In a large mixing bowl mix together the yogurt, tomato paste, paprika, ground coriander, and ½tsp of salt. Add chicken and toss to coat. Let sit at room temperature for at least 10 minutes.
3. Using a rimmed baking tray greased with 1 tbsp of oil, place the chicken on the tray, leaving space between the pieces.
4. In a bowl, mix together 1tbsp of oil, 1tsp of salt, and the pumpkin pieces. Place the pumpkin on another non-stick baking tray.
5. Place the tray with the chicken on the top rack of the oven and the pumpkin one on the lower rack. Leave to cook for about 15-20 minutes. Make sure to turn over the pumpkin after 7 minutes to ensure the pumpkin cooks through to being tender and golden brown.
6. In a blender, mix together 1/5cup of fresh lime juice, ginger, 1 cup of coriander leaves, 1/3cup of water, and 1/4cup of oil.
7. Steam enough rice to serve 2 portions, following the instructions on the rice package.
8. Divide the rice among 2 serves and top with chicken, pumpkin, and sauce. Garnish with coriander leaves

Sheet Pan Greek Lemon Chicken and Potatoes

Serves: 2
Prep: 15 minutes | **Cook:** 45 minute

Nutrition:

Cal 400 | **Fat** 25g
Carb 30g | **Protein** 35g

Ingredients:

- 2 boneless, skinless chicken breasts (about 6oz each)
- ¼ cup lemon juice (freshly squeezed)
- 2 tbsp garlic-infused olive oil
- 1 tsp dried oregano
- ½ tsp dried thyme
- ¼ tsp ground cumin
- Salt and pepper to taste
- 1 tbsp fresh parsley, chopped (optional, for garnish)
- 2 medium Yukon gold or red potatoes, cut into wedges
- 1 tbsp garlic-infused olive oil
- ½ tsp dried oregano
- Salt and pepper to taste
- Lemon wedges for serving (optional)

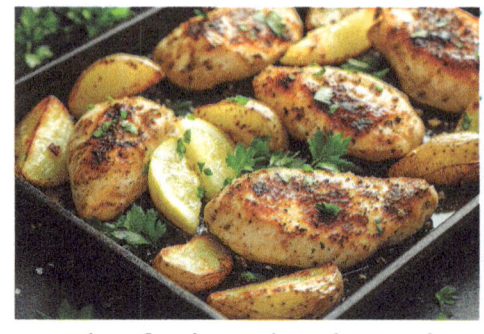

Instructions:

1. Preheat your oven to 400°F (200°C). Line a sheet pan with parchment paper or lightly grease it with olive oil.
2. In a small bowl, whisk together the lemon juice, garlic-infused olive oil, dried oregano, dried thyme, ground cumin, salt, and pepper. Place the chicken breasts in a shallow dish, and pour the marinade over them. Marinate the chicken for at least 15 minutes, or longer if you have time.
3. While the chicken is marinating, toss the potato wedges with the garlic-infused olive oil, dried oregano, salt, and pepper in a large bowl. Spread the potatoes out in an even layer on the prepared sheet pan.
4. Remove the chicken breasts from the marinade and place them on the sheet pan next to the potatoes. Discard the remaining marinade.
5. Roast in the preheated oven for 40-45 minutes, or until the chicken is cooked through (internal temperature of 165°F/74°C) and the potatoes are golden brown and crispy. Stir the potatoes halfway through cooking to ensure they cook evenly.
6. Once the chicken and potatoes are done, remove the sheet pan from the oven. Garnish the chicken with fresh parsley if desired, and serve with additional lemon wedges on the side.

Low-FODMAP Vietnamese Pho

Serves: 2
Prep: 15 minutes | **Cook:** 30 minute

Nutrition:

Cal 400 | **Fat** 8g
Carb 55g | **Protein** 25g

Ingredients:

- 4 cups chicken broth (ensure it's onion-free and garlic-free)
- 1-inch piece fresh ginger, sliced
- 1 cinnamon stick
- 2 star anise
- 2 cloves
- 1 tbsp fish sauce
- 1 tbsp soy sauce or tamari
- 1 tbsp brown sugar or maple syrup
- 4oz rice noodles
- 1 boneless, skinless chicken breast (about 6oz), thinly sliced
- ¼ cup green tops of scallions, chopped
- 1 cup bean sprouts
- ½ cup fresh cilantro, chopped
- 1 lime, cut into wedges
- Fresh basil leaves (optional)
- Fresh mint leaves (optional)
- ½ red chili, sliced (optional, adjust for spice level)

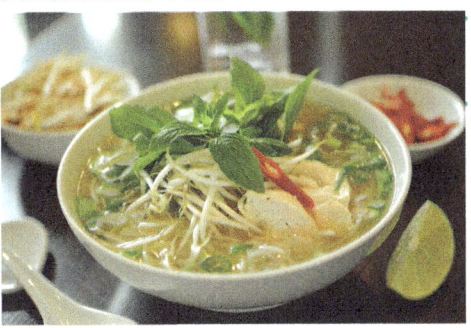

Instructions:

1. Prepare the broth. In a large pot, combine the low-FODMAP chicken broth, sliced ginger, cinnamon stick, star anise, and cloves. Bring the mixture to a boil, then reduce the heat and let it simmer for 20-30 minutes to allow the flavors to infuse.
After simmering, strain the broth to remove the ginger, cinnamon, star anise, and cloves. Return the strained broth to the pot. Stir in the fish sauce, soy sauce or tamari, and brown sugar or maple syrup. Keep the broth warm over low heat.
2. Cook the rice noodles according to the package instructions. Drain and set aside. In the same pot of broth, add the thinly sliced chicken breast and cook for 5-7 minutes, or until the chicken is fully cooked.
3. Divide the cooked rice noodles between two bowls. Ladle the hot broth and chicken over the noodles. Top each bowl with bean sprouts, green tops of scallions, fresh cilantro, basil, and mint leaves if using. Serve with lime wedges and sliced red chili on the side for added flavor.

Low-FODMAP Japanese Chicken Katsu

Serves: 2
Prep: 15 minutes | **Cook:** 20 minute

Nutrition:

Cal 550 | **Fat** 25g
Carb 55g | **Protein** 35g

Ingredients:

- 2 boneless, skinless chicken breasts (about 6oz each)
- ¼cup gluten-free flour
- 1 egg, lightly beaten
- ½cup gluten-free panko breadcrumbs
- ¼cup vegetable oil (for frying)
- Salt and pepper to taste
- 2tbsp tomato paste
- 1tbsp gluten-free soy sauce or tamari
- 1tbsp Worcestershire sauce
- 1tsp brown sugar or maple syrup
- 1tsp Dijon mustard (check for low-FODMAP ingredients)
- 1cup cooked white rice
- 1cup shredded cabbage or lettuce
- Lemon wedges (optional)

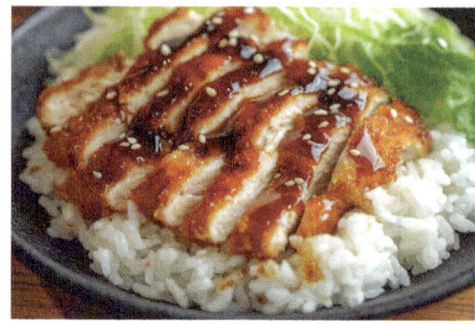

Instructions:

1. Pound the chicken breasts to an even thickness. Season both sides with salt and pepper. Set up a breading station with three shallow dishes: one with gluten-free flour, one with the beaten egg, and one with gluten-free panko breadcrumbs. Dredge each chicken breast in the flour, shaking off excess, then dip in the egg, and coat with panko breadcrumbs, pressing the breadcrumbs onto the chicken to ensure they stick well.
2. Heat vegetable oil in a large skillet over medium heat. Add the breaded chicken breasts to the skillet. Cook for 4-5 minutes per side, or until the chicken is golden brown and cooked through. The internal temperature should reach 165°F (74°C). Remove the chicken from the skillet and place it on a paper towel-lined plate to drain excess oil.
3. Prepare the Katsu Sauce. In a small bowl, whisk together the tomato paste, gluten-free soy sauce or tamari, Worcestershire sauce, brown sugar or maple syrup, and Dijon mustard until well combined. Adjust seasoning to taste.

4. Slice the chicken katsu into strips and serve over a bed of cooked white rice. Drizzle with katsu sauce and serve with shredded cabbage or lettuce on the side. Garnish with lemon wedges if desired.

Pork Lettuce Wraps

Serves: 2
Prep: 15 minutes | **Cook:** 15 minutes

Nutrition:

Cal 400 | **Fat** 25g
Carb 15g | **Protein** 20g

Ingredients:

- 8oz ground pork
- 1tbsp garlic-infused olive oil
- 1tbsp fresh ginger, grated
- 1tbsp gluten-free soy sauce or tamari
- 1tbsp rice vinegar
- 1tbsp hoisin sauce (check for low-FODMAP ingredients)
- 1tsp sesame oil
- ¼cup green tops of scallions, chopped
- ¼cup grated carrots
- ¼cup water chestnuts, chopped (optional, ensure they are low-FODMAP)
- 6-8 large lettuce leaves (e.g. butter lettuce or iceberg lettuce)
- ¼cup fresh cilantro, chopped (optional)
- ¼cup chopped peanuts (optional)
- Lime wedges for garnish

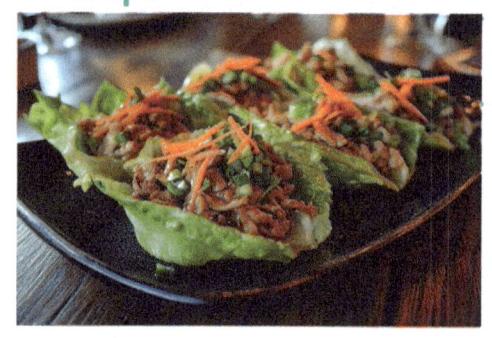

Instructions:

1. Prepare the pork filling. Heat the garlic-infused olive oil in a large skillet over medium heat. Add the grated ginger and cook for about 1 minute until fragrant. Add the ground pork to the skillet, breaking it up with a spoon as it cooks. Cook for about 5-7 minutes until the pork is browned and fully cooked through. Stir in the gluten-free soy sauce, rice vinegar, hoisin sauce, and sesame oil. Mix well to coat the pork evenly. Add the chopped green tops of scallions, grated carrots, and chopped water chestnuts (if using). Stir to combine and cook for an additional 2-3 minutes until the vegetables are slightly softened.
2. Wash and dry the lettuce leaves. Arrange them on a serving plate. Spoon the cooked pork mixture into each lettuce leaf, distributing the filling evenly.
3. Garnish the lettuce wraps with chopped fresh cilantro and peanuts if desired.
4. Serve with lime wedges on the side for an extra burst of flavor.

Beef Burger with Lactose-Free Cheese

Serves: 2
Prep: 10 minutes | **Cook:** 10 minute

Nutrition:

Cal 420 | **Fat** 25g
Carb 35g | **Protein** 25g

Ingredients:

- 9oz ground beef (80% lean)
- 2 slices lactose-free cheddar cheese
- 2 gluten-free burger buns
- 1tbsp garlic-infused olive oil (for seasoning)
- Salt and pepper to taste
- Fresh lettuce and tomato slices (within low-FODMAP limits)

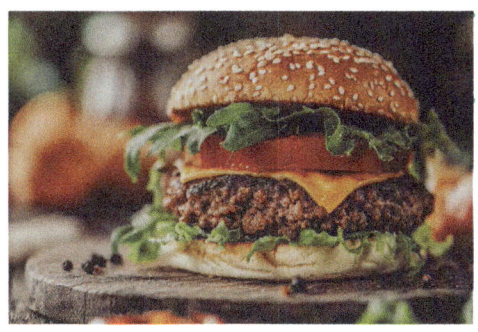

Instructions:

1. Form the ground beef into two patties.
2. Season with salt, pepper, and garlic-infused oil.
3. Cook on a grill or stovetop for about 4-5 minutes on each side.
4. Toast the buns and assemble them with lactose-free cheese, lettuce, and tomato.

Chicken Avocado Burger

Serves: 2
Prep: 10 minutes | **Cook:** 10 minute

Nutrition:

Cal 380 | **Fat** 18g
Carb 35g | **Protein** 15g

Ingredients:

- 9oz ground chicken breast
- ¼ ripe avocado (low-FODMAP portion)
- 2 gluten-free burger buns
- 1tbsp garlic-infused olive oil
- 1tbsp fresh cilantro, chopped
- Salt and pepper to taste

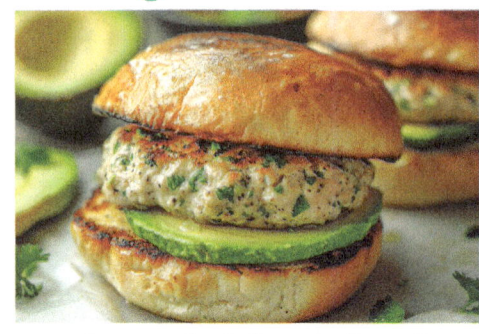

Instructions:

1. Combine ground chicken, cilantro, salt, and pepper.
2. Shape into patties and cook on a skillet for 4-5 minutes per side.
3. Top with sliced avocado and serve on toasted gluten-free buns.

Salmon Burger

Serves: 2
Prep: 15 minutes | **Cook:** 8 minutes

Nutrition:

Cal 320 | **Fat** 18g
Carb 20g | **Protein** 25g

Ingredients:

- 7oz fresh salmon fillet, finely chopped
- 1 egg (lightly beaten)
- ¼cup gluten-free breadcrumbs
- 1tsp Dijon mustard
- 1tbsp fresh dill, chopped
- Salt and pepper to taste

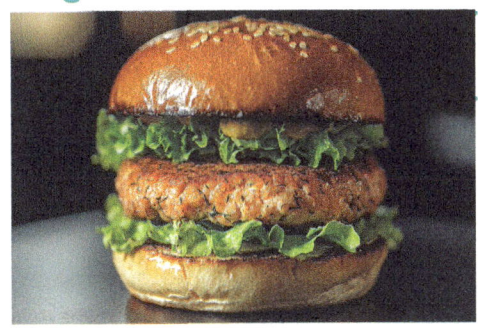

Instructions:

1. Mix salmon, egg, breadcrumbs, mustard, dill, salt, and pepper.
2. Form into two patties and refrigerate for 10 minutes.
3. Cook on a stovetop for 4 minutes per side until cooked through.

Turkey Burger with Spinach

Serves: 2
Prep: 10 minutes | **Cook:** 10 minute

Nutrition:

Cal 330 | **Fat** 15g
Carb 35g | **Protein** 30g

Ingredients:

- 9oz ground turkey breast
- ½cup fresh spinach (chopped)
- 1tbsp garlic-infused olive oil
- ½tsp cumin
- 2 gluten-free burger buns
- Salt and pepper to taste

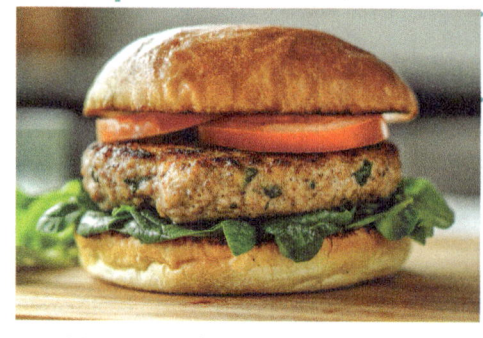

Instructions:

1. Mix ground turkey with spinach, cumin, salt, and pepper.
2. Form into patties and cook on medium heat for 5 minutes per side.
3. Serve on toasted gluten-free buns with toppings of choice.

Chapter 3: Lunch

Veggie Burger (Quinoa & Carrot)

Serves: 2
Prep: 15 minutes | **Cook:** 10 minutes

Nutrition:

Cal 280 | **Fat** 12g
Carb 35g | **Protein** 12g

Ingredients:

- ½ cup cooked quinoa
- ½ cup grated carrots
- ¼ cup gluten-free breadcrumbs
- 1 egg
- 1 tbsp garlic-infused olive oil
- ½ tsp cumin
- Salt and pepper to taste

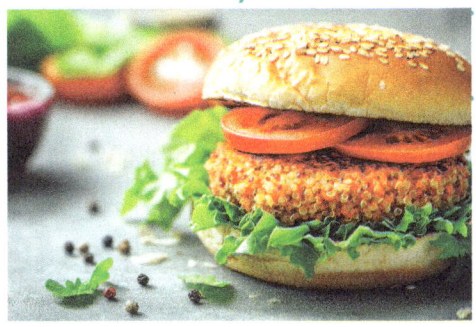

Instructions:

1. Mix quinoa, carrots, breadcrumbs, egg, cumin, salt, and pepper.
2. Form into patties and cook on medium heat for 4-5 minutes per side.
3. Serve on gluten-free buns with fresh toppings.

Chapter 4: Dinner
Salmon Bowls with Avocado and Carrot "Rice"

Serves: 2
Prep: 15 minutes | **Cook:** 20 minute

Nutrition:

Cal 475 | **Fat** 29g
Carb 16g | **Protein** 37g

Ingredients

- 3 large carrots
- 2tbsp avocado oil
- 1 pound salmon cut into fillets
- ½tsp paprika
- ½tsp ground ginger
- sea salt
- 1 bunch rainbow chard
- 1 large avocado peeled and sliced

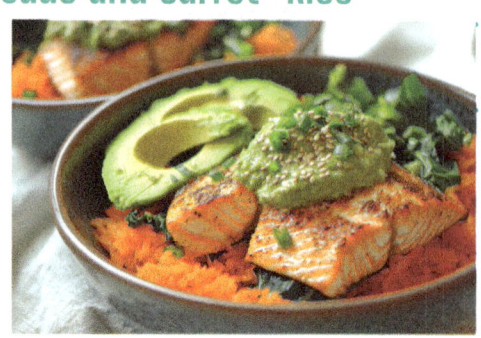

Wasabi Sauce:
- ¼cup avocado oil
- 1tbsp tahini or sunflower seed butter
- 3tbsp liquid aminos
- 2tbsp rice vinegar
- 2 to 3tsp wasabi paste to taste
- 2tsp pure maple syrup (optional)
- sea salt to taste

Instructions

1. Add all ingredients for the wasabi sauce to a blender and blend until smooth. Refrigerate the sauce until you're ready to use it.
2. Peel and chop carrots and transfer to a food processor. Pulse carrots until rice-sized pieces form. Transfer to a large saute pan with some cooking oil (like avocado oil) and saute until the carrot rice has softened and begins turning golden brown.
3. While the carrot rice is cooking, you can broil the salmon. Place oven on the high broil setting. Place the salmon fillets in a casserole dish and sprinkle with paprika, ginger, and sea salt. Broil for 10 to 15 minutes (depending on salmon thickness) on the second-from-the-top rack.
4. Add the chopped greens, a small amount of oil, and sea salt to the skillet and cook over medium until the greens have wilted. If you love garlic and onions, feel free to toss some in for flavor!
5. Divide the carrot rice, sauteed greens, salmon, and avocado between 2 bowls. Drizzle with wasabi sauce, sprinkle with chives and sesame seeds, and enjoy!

Chapter 4: Dinner

Grilled Shrimp with Lemon and Herbs

Serves: 2
Prep: 10 minutes | **Cook:** 8 minutes

Nutrition:

Cal 220 | **Fat** 16g
Carb 16g | **Protein** 37g

Ingredients:

- 9oz shrimp, peeled and deveined
- 2tbsp garlic-infused olive oil
- Juice of 1 lemon
- 1tbsp fresh parsley, chopped
- 1tbsp fresh basil, chopped
- Salt and pepper to taste

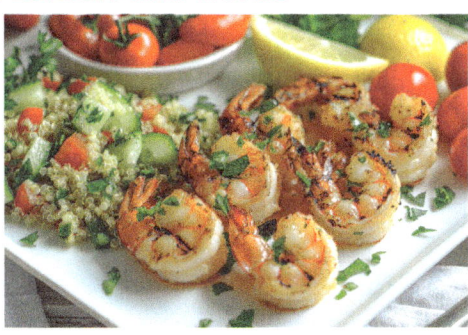

Instructions:

1. Marinate the shrimp in olive oil, lemon juice, parsley, basil, salt, and pepper for 10 minutes.
2. Grill the shrimp for 2-3 minutes on each side until pink and cooked through.
3. Serve with a quinoa salad mixed with cherry tomatoes, cucumbers, and fresh herbs.

Notes:

- The nutritional value of the dish is calculated without the side dish.

Mediterranean Baked Cod with Tomatoes and Olives

Serves: 2
Prep: 10 minutes | **Cook:** 20 minute

Nutrition:

Cal 250 | **Fat** 8g
Carb 12g | **Protein** 24g

Ingredients:

- 2 cod fillets (5oz each)
- 1cup diced tomatoes (canned or fresh)
- ¼cup green olives, sliced
- 1tbsp garlic-infused olive oil
- ½tsp dried oregano
- Salt and pepper to taste

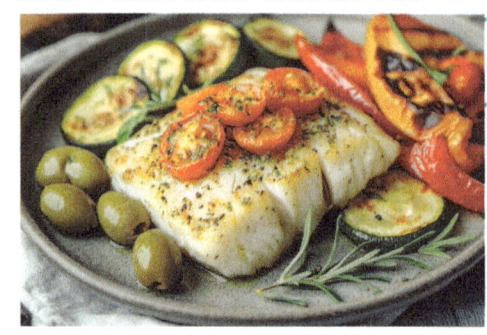

Instructions:

1. Preheat the oven to 375°F (190°C).
2. Place the cod in a baking dish, and top with tomatoes, olives, olive oil, oregano, salt, and pepper.
3. Bake for 20 minutes or until the cod is flaky.
4. Serve with roasted zucchini and bell peppers seasoned with olive oil and herbs.

Notes:

- The nutritional value of the dish is calculated without the side dish.

Mediterranean Salmon with Caper Relish

Serves: 2
Prep: 10 minutes | **Cook:** 15 minutes

Nutrition:

Cal 320 | **Fat** 22g
Carb 6g | **Protein** 28g

Ingredients:

- 2 salmon fillets (about 5oz each)
- 1tbsp garlic-infused olive oil
- 2tbsp capers, drained
- 1tbsp fresh dill, chopped
- Juice of 1 lemon
- Salt and pepper to taste

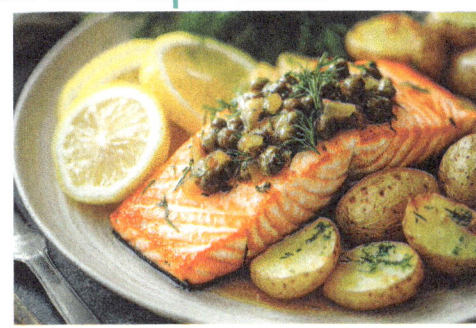

Instructions:

1. Preheat the oven to 375°F (190°C).
2. Season the salmon with olive oil, lemon juice, salt, and pepper, and bake for 12-15 minutes.
3. Top with capers and fresh dill before serving.
4. Serve with roasted baby potatoes tossed in olive oil and rosemary.

Notes:

- The nutritional value of the dish is calculated without the side dish.

Garlic-Infused Olive Oil Shrimp and Spinach Sauté

Serves: 2
Prep: 10 minutes | **Cook:** 10 minute

Nutrition:

Cal 220 | **Fat** 16g
Carb 5g | **Protein** 22g

Ingredients:

- 9oz shrimp, peeled and deveined
- 2cups fresh spinach
- 2tbsp garlic-infused olive oil
- ¼tsp red pepper flakes (optional)
- Salt and pepper to taste
- Juice of ½ lemon

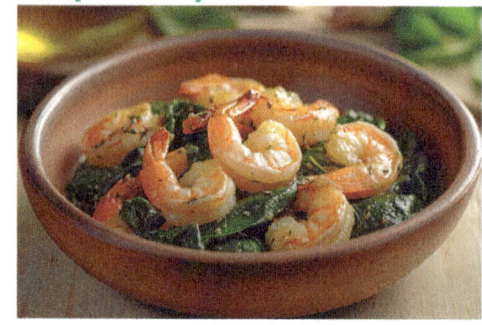

Instructions:

1. Heat olive oil in a skillet over medium heat and add the shrimp.
2. Season with salt, pepper, and red pepper flakes, and cook until pink (about 4 minutes).
3. Add spinach and cook until wilted. Drizzle with lemon juice.
4. Serve with basmati rice cooked with a bay leaf for added flavor.

Notes:

- The nutritional value of the dish is calculated without the side dish.

Chapter 4: Dinner

Orange Ginger Grilled Chicken

Serves: 2 | **Prep Time:** 10 minutes
Marinating Time: 30 minutes (optional but recommended)
Cook Time: 15-20 minutes

Nutrition:

Cal 350 | **Fat** 18g
Carb 10g | **Protein** 25g

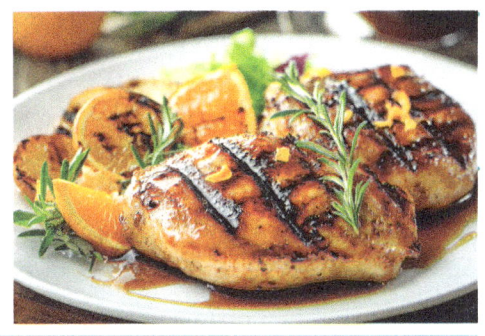

Ingredients:

- 4 boneless, skinless chicken thighs
- ¼ cup fresh orange juice
- 1 tsp orange zest
- 1 tbsp fresh ginger, grated
- 1 tbsp garlic-infused olive oil
- 1 tbsp low-sodium soy sauce (ensure it's gluten-free and low-FODMAP)
- 1 tsp maple syrup (or to taste)
- Salt and pepper to taste

Instructions:

1. In a small bowl, combine the orange juice, orange zest, grated ginger, garlic-infused olive oil, soy sauce, maple syrup, salt, and pepper. Whisk well.
2. Place the chicken thighs in a shallow dish or a resealable plastic bag. Pour the marinade over the chicken, ensuring it's well-coated. Marinate for at least 30 minutes in the refrigerator for the best flavor. If short on time, a quick 10-minute soak will still impart some flavor.
3. Preheat the grill to medium-high heat. Remove the chicken from the marinade, letting excess drip off. Discard any remaining marinade.
4. Grill the chicken for 6-8 minutes per side, or until the internal temperature reaches 165°F (75°C), and the chicken is cooked through.
5. Serve with a side of steamed jasmine rice and grilled zucchini or asparagus. The jasmine rice complements the orange-ginger flavors, while the grilled vegetables add a fresh, vibrant touch to the meal.

Notes:

- The nutritional value of the dish is calculated without the side dish.

Pumpkin Chicken Chili

Serves: 2 | **Prep Time:** 10 minutes
Cook Time: 40 minutes

Nutrition:

Cal 346 | **Fat** 11g
Carb 17g | **Protein** 36g

Ingredients:

- 1tbsp avocado oil
- 1lbs boneless skinless chicken breasts chopped
- ½tbsp chili powder
- ½tsp dried oregano
- ½tsp dried basil
- ¼tsp ground ginger
- 1/5tsp ground cinnamon
- ½tsp sea salt to taste
- ¼ green bell pepper chopped
- 1 large carrot peeled and chopped
- ½ 15-ounce can pumpkin puree
- ½cup chicken bone broth
- ½ medium heirloom tomato chopped

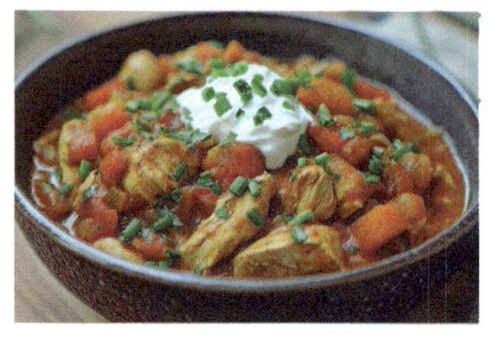

For Serving:
- coconut milk yogurt
- chives

Instructions:

1. Heat the avocado oil in a Dutch oven or stock pot over medium heat. Add the chopped chicken and brown for 3 to 5 minutes, until much liquid is seeping out (Note: if you're adding onion and garlic, do so now with the chicken!).
2. Stir in the seasonings (chili powder, oregano, basil, ginger, cinnamon, and sea salt), carrots, and bell pepper, and continue cooking from 1 to 3 minutes, until spices are fragrant.
3. Add the pumpkin puree and chicken broth, cover, and bring to a full boil. Reduce heat to a simmer and cook for 15 minutes.
4. Remove cover, add the chopped heirloom (or vine-ripened) tomato, and continue cooking at a gentle boil, stirring occasionally, until chili reaches the desired thickness, about 20 to 30 minutes.
5. Serve chili with coconut milk yogurt and chives!

Zucchini and Ground Turkey Skillet

Serves: 2 | **Prep Time:** 10 minutes
Cook Time: 20 minutes

Nutrition:

Cal 328 | **Fat** 21g
Carb 4g | **Protein** 31g

Ingredients:

- 2tbsp avocado oil
- 1lb ground turkey
- 1 medium zucchini squash chopped
- 1 1-inch ginger nub, peeled and grated
- 3 green onions chopped*
- 1 handful baby spinach
- 3 to 4tbsp coconut aminos
- 1tsp dried oregano
- 1tsp dried basil
- ¼tsp sea salt to taste

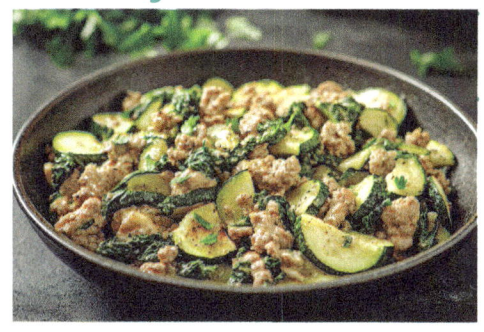

Instructions:

1. Add the avocado oil to a large skillet and heat to medium. Once the oil is hot, place the ground turkey in the skillet and brown it (keep it a brick) for 2 to 4 minutes, until it's nice and seared. Carefully flip to the other side and cook another 2 to 4 minutes.
2. Use a spatula to break up the meat into smaller pieces, then add the chopped zucchini, ginger, and green onion. Cover and cook for 2 to 3 minutes, until the zucchini begins to soften. Add the remaining ingredients and cover again for 1 to 2 minutes, until spinach has wilted.
3. Stir well and continue cooking until much of the liquid has burned off—about 3 to 4 minutes.
4. Serve it up with your favorite side dishes for the ultimate dinner.

Notes:

- *If you're very sensitive to green onion, omit it. Many people on a low-FODMAP diet can tolerate green onion (as opposed to yellow onion or red onion) but leave it out if you're unsure whether or not it works well with your system.
- The nutritional value of the dish is calculated without the side dish.

One-Skillet Ground Turkey Thai Curry with Rice

Serves: 2 | **Prep Time:** 15 minutes
Cook Time: 30 minutes

Nutrition:

Cal 542 | **Fat** 41g
Carb 41g | **Protein** 20g

Ingredients:

- ½ 15-ounce can full-fat coconut milk
- ½lb lean ground turkey
- ½tbsp fresh ginger, peeled and grated
- 1 large carrot, peeled and chopped
- ½tsp ground turmeric
- ½tsp ground paprika
- ¼tsp ground cinnamon (optional)
- 2/3cup white rice soaked for at least 1 hour
- 1cup chicken broth
- 1½tbsp coconut aminos
- ½ to 1½tbsp fish sauce to taste
- ½ medium zucchini squash chopped
- ¼tsp sea salt to taste
- ¼cup fresh basil chopped

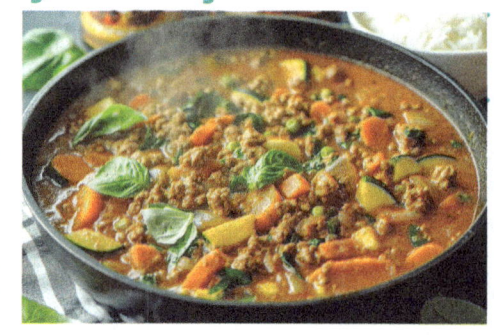

Instructions:

1. Place rice in a bowl and cover with 2 inches of water. Soak rice at least 1 hour (up to 24 hours).
2. Pour ⅓cup of coconut milk into a skillet and add the ground turkey. Brown for 3 to 4 minutes, flip to another side, and continue browning for another 2 to 3 minutes.
3. Add ginger and spices and stir, chopping up the turkey.
4. Add the carrots, remaining coconut milk, broth, coconut aminos, and fish sauce, and stir well. Stir in the rice. Cover, and bring to a full boil.
5. Reduce heat to a simmer and cook for 10 minutes.
6. Stir in the zucchini, cover, and cook an additional 10 to 15 minutes, until much of the liquid has been absorbed and the vegetables are cooked to desired doneness. Stir in the chopped basil and taste the curry. Add sea salt to taste and serve in bowls.

Chapter 4: Dinner

Mongolian Turkey

Serves: 2 | **Prep Time:** 10 minutes
Cook Time: 15 minutes

Nutrition:

Cal 300 | **Fat** 12g
Carb 18g | **Protein** 25g

Ingredients:

- 9oz ground turkey
- 1tbsp garlic-infused olive oil
- 2tbsp low-sodium soy sauce (ensure it's gluten-free and low-FODMAP)
- 2tbsp brown sugar
- ¼cup water
- 1tbsp rice vinegar
- 1tsp fresh ginger, grated
- ¼tsp red pepper flakes (optional, for a bit of spice)
- 2 green onion tops (green part only), sliced
- 1tsp sesame oil (optional, for flavor)
- Salt and pepper to taste

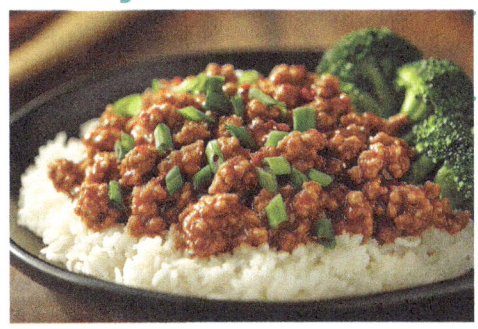

Instructions:

1. Prepare the sauce. In a small bowl, whisk together the soy sauce, brown sugar, water, and rice vinegar. Set aside.
2. Heat the garlic-infused olive oil in a large skillet over medium heat. Add the ground turkey and cook until it is browned and cooked through, breaking it into small pieces with a spatula (about 6-8 minutes). Season with salt, pepper, and add the grated ginger and red pepper flakes if desired. Cook for an additional minute.
3. Pour the sauce mixture over the cooked turkey and bring it to a simmer. Continue to cook until the sauce reduces and thickens slightly, coating the turkey (about 3-4 minutes).
4. Drizzle sesame oil over the turkey if desired, then sprinkle with sliced green onions.
5. Let the turkey rest for a couple of minutes, then plate.
6. Serve over a bed of steamed jasmine rice or quinoa with a side of steamed broccoli or snow peas to create a complete, balanced low-FODMAP meal.

Notes:

- The nutritional value of the dish is calculated without the side dish.

Turkey Meatballs with Tomato Basil Sauce

Serves: 2 | **Prep Time:** 10 minutes
Cook Time: 15 minutes

Nutrition:

Cal 280 | **Fat** 15g
Carb 12g | **Protein** 28g

Ingredients:

- 9oz ground turkey
- 1tbsp fresh basil, chopped
- 1tbsp fresh parsley, chopped
- ¼tsp dried oregano
- Salt and pepper to taste
- 1tbsp garlic-infused olive oil
- ½cup diced tomatoes (canned or fresh)

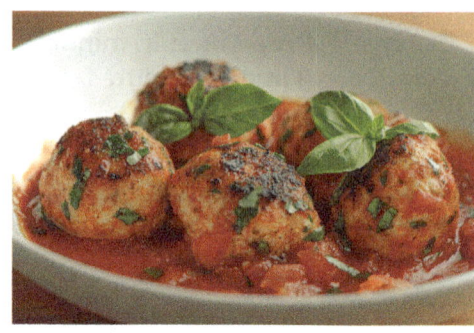

Instructions:

1. In a bowl, mix the turkey, basil, parsley, oregano, salt, and pepper. Form into meatballs.
2. Heat garlic-infused olive oil in a skillet over medium heat. Add meatballs and cook until browned.
3. Pour in diced tomatoes and simmer for 10 minutes.
4. Serve with quinoa mixed with fresh chopped spinach and a drizzle of olive oil.

Notes:

- The nutritional value of the dish is calculated without the side dish.

Lemon Herb Turkey Cutlets with Roasted Vegetables

Serves: 2 | **Prep Time:** 10 minutes
Cook Time: 20 minutes

Nutrition:

Cal 270 | **Fat** 12g
Carb 15g | **Protein** 26g

Ingredients:

- 2 turkey cutlets (about 4.5oz each)
- 1tbsp garlic-infused olive oil
- Juice and zest of 1 lemon
- 1tbsp fresh rosemary, chopped
- Salt and pepper to taste
- 1cup zucchini and bell peppers, sliced

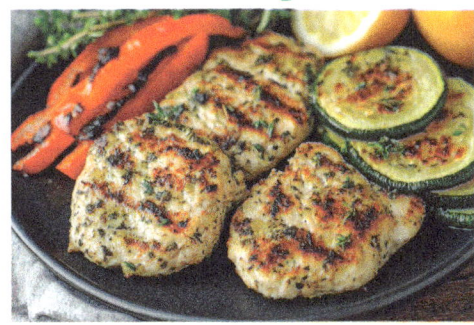

Instructions:

1. Rub the turkey cutlets with olive oil, lemon juice, zest, rosemary, salt, and pepper.
2. Grill or pan-sear the turkey cutlets for 4-5 minutes per side, or until cooked through.
3. Roast the zucchini and bell peppers at 400°F (200°C) for 15-20 minutes until tender.
4. Serve with steamed jasmine rice.

Notes:

- The nutritional value of the dish is calculated without the side dish.

Turkey Stuffed Bell Peppers

Serves: 2 | **Prep Time:** 10 minutes
Cook Time: 25 minutes

Nutrition:

Cal 300 | **Fat** 12g
Carb 20g | **Protein** 22g

Ingredients:

- 9oz ground turkey
- ½cup cooked quinoa
- 2 large bell peppers, halved and seeds removed
- 1tbsp garlic-infused olive oil
- 1tbsp fresh parsley, chopped
- Salt and pepper to taste

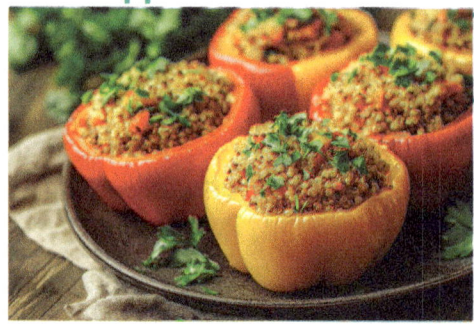

Instructions:

1. In a skillet, cook ground turkey with olive oil until browned. Season with salt, pepper, and parsley.
2. Stir in the cooked quinoa and remove from heat.
3. Stuff the bell pepper halves with the turkey mixture and bake at 375°F (190°C) for 20-25 minutes.

Chapter 4: Dinner

Turkey Patties with Olive Tapenade

Serves: 2 | **Prep Time:** 10 minutes
Cook Time: 15 minutes

Nutrition:

Cal 280 | **Fat** 18g
Carb 12g | **Protein** 23g

Ingredients:

- 9oz ground turkey
- 1tbsp garlic-infused olive oil
- 1tbsp chopped fresh basil
- Salt and pepper to taste
- ¼cup chopped olives
- 1tbsp capers
- 1tbsp fresh parsley, chopped

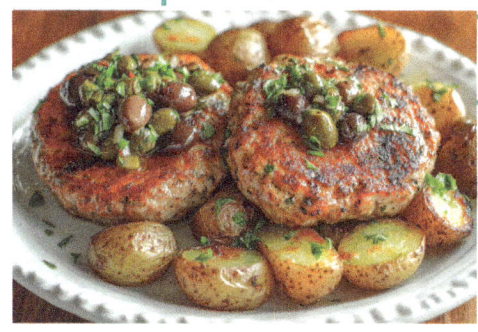

Instructions:

1. Mix ground turkey with basil, salt, and pepper. Form into patties.
2. Heat olive oil in a skillet over medium heat. Cook the patties for 6-7 minutes per side, or until cooked through.
3. Combine olives, capers, and parsley for a quick tapenade. Spoon over the cooked patties.
4. Serve with roasted baby potatoes seasoned with rosemary and olive oil.

Notes:

- The nutritional value of the dish is calculated without the side dish.

Basil Coconut Milk Ground Beef Skillet

Serves: 2 | **Prep Time:** 15 minutes
Cook Time: 25 minutes

Nutrition:

Cal 420 | **Fat** 24g
Carb 40g | **Protein** 24g

Ingredients:

For the Basil Coconut Milk Sauce:
- ½cup fresh basil, tightly packed
- ½ can (200 ml) coconut milk (ensure no additives, check for low-FODMAP compliance)
- 1tbsp fresh ginger, grated
- 1tbsp fresh lemongrass, minced (or substitute with 1tsp lemon zest for low-FODMAP)
- 1 ½tbsp coconut aminos
- 1tbsp lime juice (or rice vinegar)
- ½tsp sea salt

For the Ground Beef Skillet:
- 1cup cooked jasmine rice (or use soaked and drained white rice)
- 1tbsp garlic-infused olive oil or avocado oil
- ½lb grass-fed ground beef
- 1 large carrot, peeled and chopped
- 1cup low-FODMAP chicken or beef broth (check for no onion or garlic ingredients)
- 1cup broccoli florets (stick to low-FODMAP portion)
- ¼ red bell pepper, cut into matchsticks

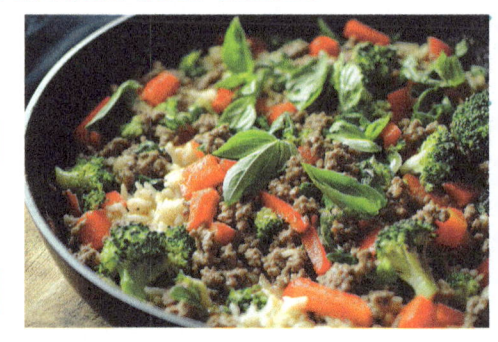

Instructions:

1. If soaking the rice, place it in water for at least 30 minutes before cooking. Drain and set aside when ready to use.
2. Make the Basil Coconut Sauce. In a blender, combine the fresh basil, coconut milk, grated ginger, lemongrass (or lemon zest), coconut aminos, lime juice, and sea salt. Blend until smooth. Set aside.
3. Cook the Beef. Heat the garlic-infused oil in a large skillet over medium heat. Add the ground beef and cook for about 5 minutes, breaking it up as it browns. Season with a pinch of salt and pepper if desired.
4. Stir the soaked rice, chopped carrots, basil coconut sauce, and broth into the skillet. Bring the mixture to a gentle boil, then reduce heat to a simmer. Cover and cook for 10 minutes.

5. Add the broccoli florets and red bell pepper to the skillet. Stir well, cover, and continue cooking for another 10 minutes, or until the liquid has been absorbed and the vegetables are tender.
6. Remove from heat and let sit for a few minutes before serving. Dish up into bowls and enjoy!

Spiced Beef Patties with Cucumber Yogurt Sauce

Serves: 2 | **Prep Time:** 10 minutes
Cook Time: 10 minutes

Nutrition:

Cal 300 | **Fat** 18g
Carb 10g | **Protein** 25g

Ingredients:

- 9oz ground beef
- 1tsp ground cumin
- ½tsp ground coriander
- 1tbsp fresh parsley, chopped
- Salt and pepper to taste
- 1tbsp garlic-infused olive oil
- ¼cup lactose-free Greek yogurt
- ¼ cucumber, grated and squeezed dry
- 1tsp fresh mint, chopped

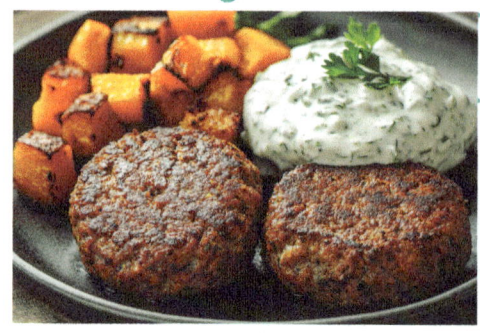

Instructions:

1. In a bowl, combine the ground beef, cumin, coriander, parsley, salt, and pepper. Form into patties.
2. Heat garlic-infused olive oil in a skillet and cook patties for about 4-5 minutes per side, until cooked through.
3. In a small bowl, mix the Greek yogurt, grated cucumber, and mint to make the sauce. Serve the patties with a dollop of the sauce.
4. Serve with roasted butternut squash cubes. Toss the squash with a little olive oil and fresh thyme, then roast until caramelized. The sweetness and soft texture contrast nicely with the beef patties.

Notes:

- The nutritional value of the dish is calculated without the side dish.

Chapter 4: Dinner

Beef and Tomato Stir-Fry with Fresh Basil

Serves: 2 | **Prep Time:** 10 minutes
Cook Time: 10 minutes

Nutrition:

Cal 270 | **Fat** 16g
Carb 10g | **Protein** 27g

Ingredients:

- 9oz beef sirloin, thinly sliced
- 1tbsp garlic-infused olive oil
- ½cup cherry tomatoes, halved
- 1tbsp low-sodium soy sauce (gluten-free)
- 1tbsp fresh basil, chopped
- Salt and pepper to taste

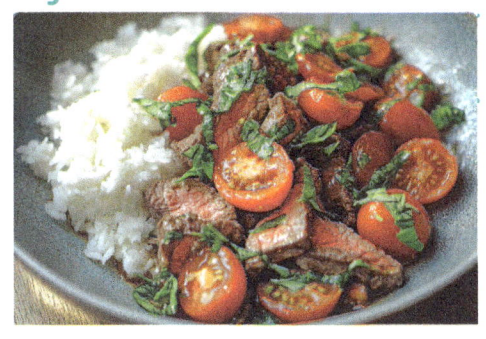

Instructions:

1. Heat garlic-infused olive oil in a skillet over medium heat. Add the beef and cook for 3-4 minutes, until browned.
2. Add the cherry tomatoes, soy sauce, salt, and pepper. Stir-fry for another 3-4 minutes until the tomatoes soften.
3. Stir in fresh basil just before serving.
4. Serve with a side of steamed jasmine rice for a balanced meal.

Notes:

- The nutritional value of the dish is calculated without the side dish.

Creamy Vegan Mushroom Soup

Serves: 2 | **Prep Time:** 20 minutes
Cook Time: 1 hour

Nutrition:

Cal 404 | **Fat** 19g
Carb 45g | **Protein** 17g

Ingredients

- ¼ cup raw cashews soaked
- ½ tbsp avocado oil
- ½ small yellow onion diced
- 2 cloves of garlic minced
- ½ large carrot peeled and chopped
- ½ lb baby portobello mushrooms
- ½ cup wild rice
- 3 cups vegetable broth*
- ½ tsp sea salt to taste
- 1 tsp dried oregano
- ½ tsp dried rosemary
- ½ cup full-fat canned coconut milk
- 1 tbsp nutritional yeast
- ½ tsp cider vinegar or lemon juice

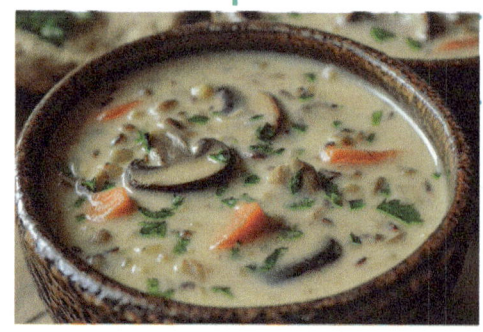

Instructions

1. Place cashews in a bowl and cover with water. Soak at least 1 hour, up to 8 hours. Strain and set aside until ready to use.
2. Heat the avocado oil in a Dutch oven or large stock pot over medium-high. Add the onion and sauté, stirring occasionally, until the onion begins turning brown, about 8 minutes.
3. Add the carrot, garlic, and mushrooms, and continue cooking, stirring occasionally, until mushrooms begin to deepen in color, about 5 minutes.
4. Add the rice, vegetable broth, sea salt, oregano, and nutritional yeast. Cover and bring to a full boil.
5. While the soup is coming to a boil, blend the coconut milk and cashews together in a small blender. Stir this mixture into the pot, replace the cover, and reduce heat to medium-low to cook at a simmer. Continue cooking until soup has thickened and rice is cooked through, about 45 minutes. Taste the soup for flavor and add more sea salt according to taste.
6. Scoop soup into bowls and serve!

Notes:

- Use beef bone broth or chicken broth instead of vegetable broth if you aren't vegan.

Shredded Brussels Sprout Salad with Roasted Sweet Potatoes

Serves: 2 | **Prep Time:** 15 minutes
Cook Time: 25 minutes

Nutrition:

Cal 500 | **Fat** 34g
Carb 42g | **Protein** 11g

Ingredients:

For the Roasted Sweet Potato:
- 1 medium sweet potato, chopped into bite-sized pieces
- 1 tbsp avocado oil
- Pinch of sea salt

For the Brussels Sprout Salad:
- ½lb Brussels sprouts, shredded or thinly sliced
- ½cup fresh blueberries or raspberries (low-FODMAP substitute for dried cranberries)
- 2tbsp crumbled feta cheese (optional, or omit for dairy-free)
- ¼cup raw pecans, chopped
- ½tbsp maple syrup (optional, for lightly glazing pecans)

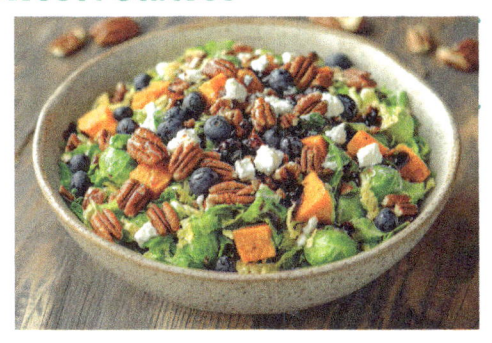

For the Cinnamon Balsamic Vinaigrette:
- 2tbsp olive oil
- 2tbsp balsamic vinegar
- 1tbsp pure maple syrup
- A pinch of ground cinnamon
- Salt to taste

Instructions:

1. Preheat the oven to 400°F (200°C). Place the sweet potato cubes on a baking sheet, drizzle with avocado oil, and season with a pinch of sea salt. Toss to coat. Bake for 20-25 minutes, stirring halfway through, until golden brown and tender. Set aside to cool.
2. In a small bowl, whisk together olive oil, balsamic vinegar, maple syrup, cinnamon, and salt. Set aside.
3. Toast the pecans (optional). In a small pan over medium heat, toast the chopped pecans for about 3 minutes, stirring occasionally. Optionally, add ½tbsp maple syrup to lightly glaze the pecans. Remove from heat and let it cool.
4. Rinse and pat dry the Brussels sprouts. Using a sharp knife, food processor, or mandoline, thinly slice the Brussels sprouts. Transfer them to a large bowl.

5. Add the roasted sweet potatoes, blueberries or raspberries, crumbled feta cheese (if using), and toasted pecans to the Brussels sprouts. Toss to combine. Pour the balsamic vinaigrette over the salad, and toss until everything is evenly coated.
6. Taste and adjust seasoning with more salt if needed.

Vegan Mexican Black Bean and Sweet Potato Skillet

Serves: 2 | **Prep Time:** 15 minutes
Cook Time: 25 minutes

Nutrition:

Cal 145 | **Fat** 3g
Carb 25g | **Protein** 14g

Ingredients:

- 1tbsp garlic-infused olive oil (for low-FODMAP flavor)
- 1 red bell pepper, cored and chopped
- 1cup uncooked quinoa, soaked for 15 minutes and drained
- 1½cups low-FODMAP vegetable broth or water
- ½cup low-FODMAP salsa (check ingredients for no onion or garlic)
- 1tbsp chili powder
- ½tsp ground cumin
- 1tsp sea salt (to taste)
- 1 medium sweet potato, peeled and cut into 1-inch cubes
- ½cup canned lentils, drained and rinsed (substitute for black beans to keep it low-FODMAP)

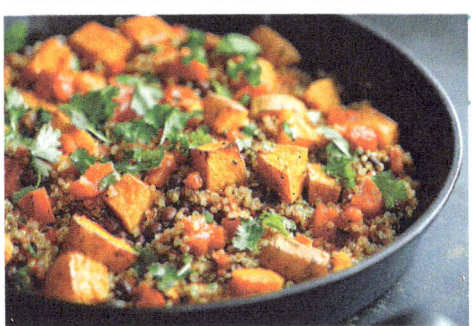

Instructions:

1. Place the quinoa in a bowl, cover it with water, and let it soak for at least 15 minutes. Drain and set aside.
2. In a large skillet or Dutch oven, heat the garlic-infused olive oil over medium heat. Add the red bell pepper and sauté for 3 minutes, stirring occasionally, until the pepper is slightly softened.
3. Add the drained quinoa, vegetable broth, salsa, chili powder, cumin, and sea salt to the skillet. Stir well and bring the mixture to a boil. Reduce the heat to a simmer, cover, and cook for 5 minutes.
4. Add the sweet potato cubes and drained lentils to the skillet. Stir well, cover again, and continue cooking for 10-15 minutes, until the quinoa and sweet potatoes are tender and the liquid is absorbed.
5. Remove the skillet from heat, and taste for seasoning. Add more salt, salsa, or a squeeze of lime juice to taste, if desired.

Chapter 5: Desserts

Berry Frangipane Tart

Serves: 6
Prep: 10 minutes | **Cook:** 30 minute

Nutrition:

Cal 274 | **Fat** 19g
Carb 24g | **Protein** 4g

Ingredients:

- 2.5oz butter, softened
- ½tsp vanilla extract
- ⅓cup caster sugar
- 1 egg
- ¾cup almond meal
- 1tbsp gluten-free corn flour
- 5oz blueberries (or a mix of low-FODMAP berries)
- 2tbsp pure icing sugar

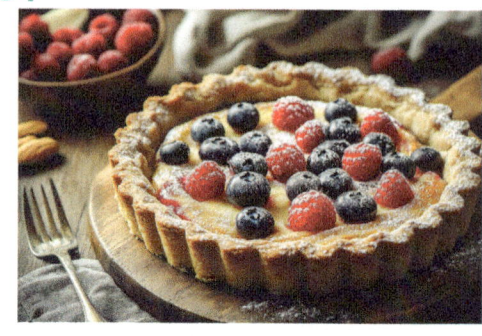

Instructions:

1. Preheat oven to 180°C/356°F. Grease 6-8 loose-based flan tins and place on oven tray. You can also use one large loose-based shallow tin.
2. Mix butter, vanilla, and caster sugar together in a small bowl with an electric mixer until combined. Add the egg and mix well.
3. Gently mix in the almond meal and corn flour, and stir until smooth. Spoon the mixture into the tins, smooth the surface with the back of a hot spoon, and sprinkle with blueberries, pushing them into the mix slightly.
4. Bake in the oven for 30 min until the surface is golden brown and firm to touch. Let stand before turning out of the trays.
5. Serve with a dusting of icing sugar.

Lemon & Blueberry Cheesecake Slice

Serves: 12 | **Prep:** 15 minutes
Cook: 4 hours 30 minutes

Nutrition:

Cal 189 | **Fat** 9g
Carb 21g | **Protein** 6g

Ingredients:

- 7oz sweet plain biscuits
- 2tbsp butter, melted
- 9oz reduced-fat cream cheese (lactose-free if required)
- 7oz plain lactose-free yogurt
- ⅓cup caster sugar
- 2tbsp lemon juice
- Zest of 1 lemon
- 1tsp vanilla extract
- 0.35oz corn flour (cornstarch)
- 2 egg whites
- 1cup fresh blueberries or raspberries (can use frozen)

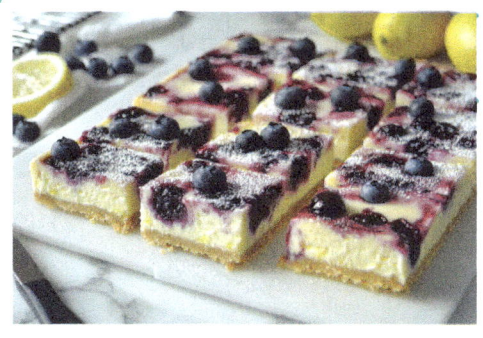

Instructions:

1. Preheat oven to 180°C (350°F) and line an 8x8 inch slice tray with baking paper, leaving some paper overhanging on the sides.
2. Add the sweet plain biscuits to a food processor and pulse until they form a fine crumb. Add melted butter and pulse again until the mixture comes together. Pour the mixture into the prepared slice tray and press down firmly using your hands or the back of a spoon. Bake in the oven for 10 minutes or until lightly golden and then set aside to cool.
3. Using a hand/stand mixer or food processor, beat cream cheese and yogurt together until smooth and well combined. Next, beat in caster sugar, lemon juice, zest, vanilla extract, corn flour, and egg whites (add one at a time). Continue to beat until the mixture is light, fluffy, and well combined.
4. Finally, gently stir through the berries until just combined.
5. Pour the filling over the prepared base and bake in the oven at 180°C (350°F) for approximately 25-30 minutes.
6. Remove cheesecake from the oven and set aside to cool for 30 minutes or so before transferring to the fridge. Refrigerate for at least 4 hours (preferably overnight) before serving.
7. Cut cheesecake into bars to serve!

Clafoutis Cake

Serves: 4
Prep: 10 minutes | **Cook:** 40 minute

Nutrition:

Cal 220 | **Fat** 10g
Carb 28g | **Protein** 7g

Ingredients:

- ½ cup lactose-free milk
- ¼ cup lactose-free cream
- 3 large eggs
- ¼ cup gluten-free flour
- ¼ cup granulated sugar
- 1 tsp vanilla extract
- ¼ tsp salt
- 1 cup mixed low-FODMAP berries (such as strawberries, raspberries, or blueberries)
- 1 tbsp powdered sugar for dusting (optional)

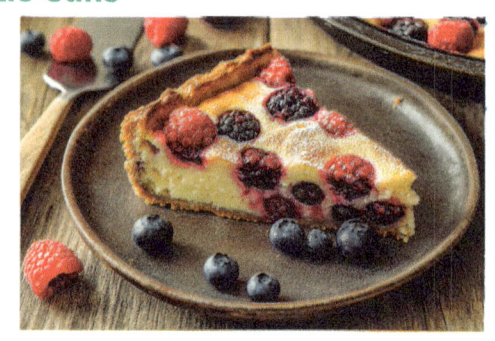

Instructions:

1. Preheat your oven to 350°F (180°C). Grease a 9-inch pie dish or baking dish with butter or cooking spray.
2. In a mixing bowl, whisk together the eggs and sugar until well combined and slightly frothy. Add the gluten-free flour, salt, and vanilla extract, and whisk until smooth. Gradually whisk in the lactose-free milk and cream until you have a smooth batter.
3. Spread the berries evenly across the bottom of the greased pie dish. Pour the batter over the berries, ensuring they are evenly distributed.
4. Bake in the preheated oven for 35-40 minutes, or until the Clafoutis is puffed, golden brown, and set in the center. The edges should be slightly browned, and a toothpick inserted into the center should come out clean.
5. Remove from the oven and let it cool slightly. Serve warm or at room temperature.

Banana Bars

Serves: 8
Prep: 15 minutes | **Cook:** 30 minute

Nutrition:

Cal 350 | **Fat** 15g
Carb 45g | **Protein** 4g

Ingredients:

For the Banana Bars:
- 1cup mashed ripe bananas (about 2 medium bananas)
- ¼cup lactose-free butter, softened
- ½cup granulated sugar
- 1 large egg
- 1tsp vanilla extract
- 1cup gluten-free all-purpose flour
- ½tsp baking soda
- ¼tsp salt

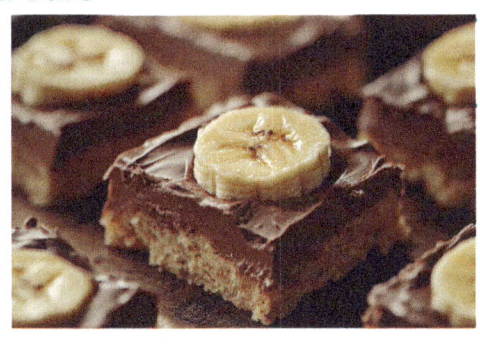

For the Chocolate Cream Cheese Frosting:
- 4oz lactose-free cream cheese, softened
- 2tbsp lactose-free butter, softened
- ¼cup cocoa powder
- ½tsp vanilla extract
- 1½cups powdered sugar

Instructions:

1. Preheat your oven to 350°F (180°C). Grease a 9x9-inch baking dish or line it with parchment paper.
2. In a large mixing bowl, beat together the lactose-free butter and sugar until light and fluffy. Add the egg and vanilla extract, and beat until well combined. Mix in the mashed bananas until smooth.
   In a separate bowl, whisk together the gluten-free flour, baking soda, and salt. Gradually add the dry ingredients to the wet ingredients, mixing until just combined. Pour the batter into the prepared baking dish and spread it evenly.
3. Bake the Banana Bars in the preheated oven for 25-30 minutes, or until a toothpick inserted into the center comes out clean. Allow the bars to cool completely in the baking dish.
4. Prepare the Chocolate Cream Cheese Frosting. In a mixing bowl, beat the lactose-free cream cheese and butter until smooth. Add the cocoa powder and vanilla extract, and beat until combined. Gradually add the powdered sugar, mixing until smooth and creamy.
5. Once the banana bars are completely cool, spread the chocolate cream cheese frosting evenly over the top. Cut into squares and serve.

Lemon Cream Pie Bars

Serves: 12
Prep: 20 minutes | **Cook:** 30 minute

Nutrition:

Cal 220 | **Fat** 11g
Carb 28g | **Protein** 4g

Ingredients:

For the Crust:
- 1 cup gluten-free graham cracker crumbs
- ¼ cup lactose-free butter, melted
- 2 tbsp granulated sugar

For the Lemon Filling:
- 4 large egg yolks
- 1 can (14oz) sweetened condensed lactose-free milk
- ½ cup fresh lemon juice (about 2-3 lemons)
- 1 tbsp lemon zest

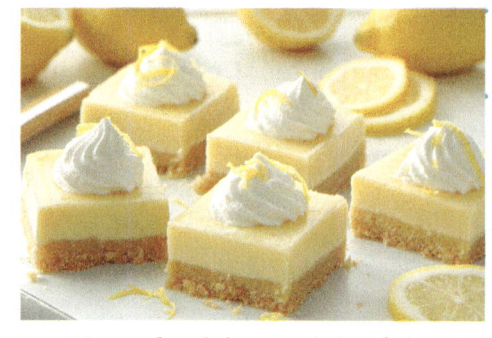

For the Topping (optional):
- ½ cup lactose-free whipped cream
- Fresh lemon slices or zest for garnish

Instructions:

1. Preheat your oven to 350°F (180°C). Grease an 8x8-inch baking pan or line it with parchment paper. In a mixing bowl, combine the gluten-free graham cracker crumbs, melted lactose-free butter, and granulated sugar. Press the mixture evenly into the bottom of the prepared baking pan. Bake the crust in the preheated oven for 8-10 minutes, or until lightly golden. Remove from the oven and let it cool slightly.
2. In a medium bowl, whisk together the egg yolks, lactose-free sweetened condensed milk, fresh lemon juice, and lemon zest until smooth and well combined. Pour the lemon mixture over the baked crust, spreading it evenly.
3. Return the pan to the oven and bake for 15-20 minutes, or until the filling is set and slightly firm to the touch. Remove from the oven and let the bars cool to room temperature. Then refrigerate for at least 2 hours to fully set.
4. Once set, remove the bars from the pan and cut them into squares. Top with lactose-free whipped cream and garnish with lemon slices or additional lemon zest if desired.
5. Serve chilled.

Tiramisu

Serves: 8 | **Prep:** 25 minutes
Chill Time: 4-6 hours (or overnight

Nutrition:

Cal 300 | **Fat** 20g
Carb 35g | **Protein** 7g

Ingredients:

For the Ladyfingers:
- ½cup gluten-free flour
- 3 large eggs, separated
- ¼cup granulated sugar
- ¼tsp vanilla extract
- ¼tsp salt

For the Mascarpone Filling:
- 8oz lactose-free mascarpone cheese
- ½cup lactose-free heavy cream
- ¼cup powdered sugar
- 1tsp vanilla extract

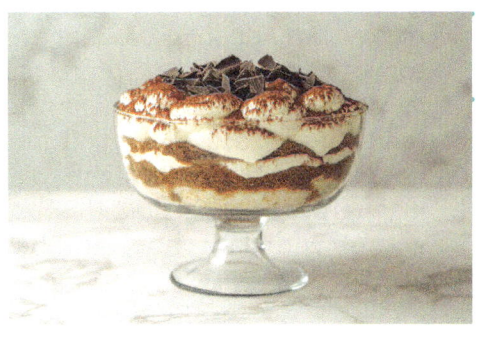

For the Coffee Mixture:
- 1cup brewed espresso or strong coffee, cooled
- 2tbsp maple syrup or granulated sugar (optional, for sweetness)
- 1tbsp coffee liqueur (optional but adds depth)

For Dusting:
- 2tbsp unsweetened cocoa powder
- Dark chocolate shavings (optional, for garnish)

Instructions:

1. Prepare the Gluten-Free Ladyfingers.
   Preheat your oven to 350°F (180°C) and line a baking sheet with parchment paper. In a bowl, beat the egg whites with salt until soft peaks form. Gradually add half the sugar, beating until stiff peaks form. In another bowl, beat the egg yolks with the remaining sugar until pale and thick. Fold in the gluten-free flour and vanilla extract. Gently fold the egg whites into the yolk mixture until combined. Transfer the batter to a piping bag and pipe fingers onto the prepared baking sheet. Bake for 10-12 minutes, or until lightly golden. Allow to cool.
2. Prepare the Mascarpone Filling.
   In a large mixing bowl, beat the lactose-free mascarpone cheese until smooth. In a separate bowl, whip the lactose-free heavy cream with powdered sugar and vanilla extract until soft peaks form. Gently fold the whipped cream into the mascarpone until combined and smooth.

3. Assemble the Tiramisu.
   Dip each ladyfinger into the cooled coffee mixture, ensuring they are soaked but not soggy. Arrange a layer of soaked ladyfingers at the bottom of a serving dish. Spread half of the mascarpone mixture over the ladyfingers. Repeat with another layer of soaked ladyfingers and the remaining mascarpone mixture. Cover and refrigerate for at least 4-6 hours, preferably overnight, to allow the flavors to meld.
4. Just before serving, dust the top with unsweetened cocoa powder and garnish with dark chocolate shavings if desired. Slice and serve chilled.

Chapter 5: Desserts

Chocolate Truffles

Serves: 12
Prep: 15 minutes | **Chill Time:** 2 hour

Nutrition:

Cal 110 | **Fat** 8g
Carb 10g | **Protein** 2g

Ingredients:

- 8oz dark chocolate (ensure it's at least 70% cocoa)
- ½ cup lactose-free heavy cream
- 1 tsp vanilla extract
- 2 tbsp lactose-free butter
- ¼ cup unsweetened cocoa powder (for rolling)
- Optional: finely chopped nuts, shredded coconut, or crushed low-FODMAP cookies for rolling

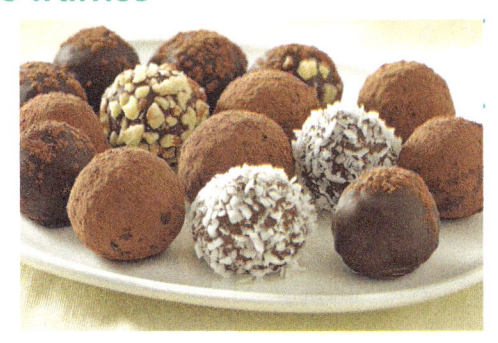

Instructions:

1. Prepare the Ganache.
2. Chop the low-FODMAP dark chocolate into small pieces and place it in a heatproof bowl.
   In a small saucepan, heat the lactose-free heavy cream over medium heat until it just begins to simmer (do not let it boil). Pour the hot cream over the chopped chocolate and let it sit for about 2 minutes. Add the vanilla extract and lactose-free butter to the mixture, then gently stir until the chocolate is fully melted and the mixture is smooth and glossy.
3. Cover the bowl with plastic wrap and refrigerate the ganache for at least 2 hours, or until it is firm enough to shape.
4. Shape the Truffles.
   Once the ganache is firm, use a small spoon or melon baller to scoop out portions of the mixture.
   Roll each portion into a ball using your hands. Work quickly to avoid melting the chocolate.
5. Place the unsweetened cocoa powder (or other desired coatings) in a shallow dish. Roll each truffle in the cocoa powder until fully coated.
6. Transfer the truffles to a serving dish or an airtight container. Store in the refrigerator until ready to serve.

Pineapple Upside-Down Cake

Serves: 8
Prep: 20 minutes | **Cook:** 40 minute

Nutrition:

Cal 320 | **Fat** 15g
Carb 45g | **Protein** 4g

Ingredients:

For the Topping:
- ¼cup lactose-free butter, melted
- ½cup brown sugar, packed
- 1 can (8oz) pineapple slices in juice (ensure no added sugar or high-FODMAP ingredients)
- Maraschino cherries (optional)

For the Cake:
- 1½cups gluten-free all-purpose flour
- ½cup granulated sugar
- ½cup lactose-free butter, softened
- 2 large eggs
- ½cup lactose-free milk
- 1tsp vanilla extract
- 1tsp baking powder
- ¼tsp salt

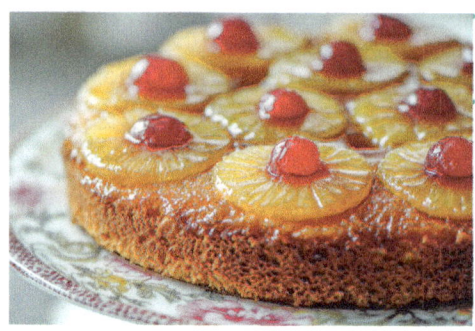

Instructions:

1. Preheat your oven to 350°F (180°C).
   Pour the melted lactose-free butter into the bottom of a 9-inch round cake pan, spreading it evenly.
   Sprinkle the brown sugar over the melted butter. Arrange the pineapple slices on top of the sugar layer. If using, place a maraschino cherry in the center of each pineapple ring.
2. In a mixing bowl, cream the lactose-free butter and granulated sugar together until light and fluffy. Beat in the eggs one at a time, followed by the vanilla extract. In a separate bowl, whisk together the gluten-free flour, baking powder, and salt. Gradually add the dry ingredients to the wet mixture, alternating with the lactose-free milk, until the batter is smooth.
3. Pour the cake batter over the pineapple and sugar layer in the cake pan, spreading it evenly.
   Bake in the preheated oven for 35-40 minutes, or until a toothpick inserted into the center comes out clean. Allow the cake to cool in the pan for about 10 minutes before carefully inverting it onto a serving plate.
4. Slice and serve the cake warm or at room temperature.

Chocolate Cake

Serves: 8
Prep: 15 minutes | **Cook:** 30 minute

Nutrition:

Cal 350 | **Fat** 12g
Carb 50g | **Protein** 4g

Ingredients:

For the Cake:
- 1cup gluten-free all-purpose flour
- ½cup cocoa powder
- 1cup granulated sugar
- 1tsp baking powder
- ½tsp baking soda
- ¼tsp salt
- ½cup lactose-free milk
- ¼cup lactose-free yogurt
- ¼cup vegetable oil
- 2 large eggs
- 1tsp vanilla extract
- ½cup hot water

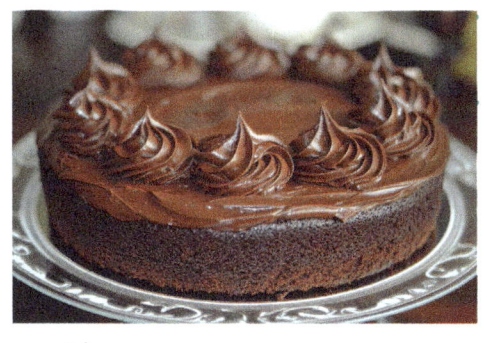

For the Frosting:
- ½cup lactose-free butter, softened
- ¼cup cocoa powder
- 1½cups powdered sugar
- ¼cup lactose-free milk
- 1tsp vanilla extract

Instructions:

1. Prepare the Cake Batter.
   Preheat your oven to 350°F (180°C). Grease and flour an 8-inch round cake pan or line it with parchment paper. In a large mixing bowl, sift together the gluten-free flour, cocoa powder, sugar, baking powder, baking soda, and salt. Add the lactose-free milk, yogurt, vegetable oil, eggs, and vanilla extract. Beat the mixture on medium speed until well combined. Gradually add the hot water, mixing on low speed until the batter is smooth. The batter will be thin.
2. Pour the batter into the prepared cake pan.
   Bake in the preheated oven for 25-30 minutes, or until a toothpick inserted into the center comes out clean. Allow the cake to cool in the pan for 10 minutes before transferring it to a wire rack to cool completely.
3. Prepare the frosting.
   In a medium bowl, beat the lactose-free butter until creamy. Gradually add the cocoa powder and powdered sugar, mixing on low speed. Add

the lactose-free milk and vanilla extract, and beat until the frosting is smooth and spreadable. Once the cake is completely cool, frost the top and sides of the cake as desired.
4. Slice and serve the cake. Store any leftovers in an airtight container.

Blueberry Cobbler

Serves: 6
Prep: 15 minutes | **Cook:** 30 minute

Nutrition:

Cal 250 | **Fat** 8g
Carb 45g | **Protein** 2g

Ingredients:

For the Blueberry Filling:
- 3 cups fresh or frozen blueberries
- ¼ cup granulated sugar
- 1 tbsp cornstarch
- 1 tbsp fresh lemon juice
- 1 tsp lemon zest (optional)

For the Cobbler Topping:
- 1 cup gluten-free all-purpose flour
- ¼ cup granulated sugar
- 1 tsp baking powder
- ¼ tsp salt
- ¼ cup lactose-free butter, cold and cut into small pieces
- ½ cup lactose-free milk
- 1 tsp vanilla extract

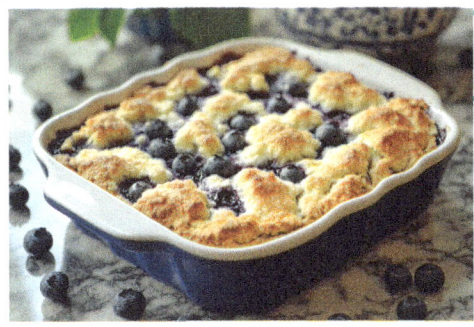

Instructions:

1. Preheat your oven to 375°F (190°C). Lightly grease a 9-inch baking dish or pie dish.
2. In a large bowl, combine the blueberries, granulated sugar, cornstarch, lemon juice, and lemon zest (if using). Toss until the blueberries are evenly coated. Pour the blueberry mixture into the prepared baking dish and spread it out evenly.
3. Prepare the cobbler topping. In a separate bowl, whisk together the gluten-free flour, granulated sugar, baking powder, and salt. Add the cold, diced lactose-free butter to the flour mixture and use a pastry cutter or your fingers to work the butter into the flour until the mixture resembles coarse crumbs. Stir in the lactose-free milk and vanilla extract until just combined. The dough will be thick and sticky.
4. Drop spoonfuls of the cobbler dough over the blueberry filling. The dough doesn't need to cover the blueberries completely; it will spread as it bakes.

5. Bake the cobbler in the preheated oven for 25-30 minutes, or until the topping is golden brown and the blueberry filling is bubbling. Remove from the oven and let it cool for a few minutes before serving.
6. Serve the blueberry cobbler warm, optionally with a scoop of lactose-free vanilla ice cream or a dollop of lactose-free whipped cream.

Chapter 6: Practical Tips and Recommendations

A Guide to Reading Ingredient Labels on a Low-FODMAP Diet

While the only reliable way to know the exact FODMAP content of a food product is through lab testing, checking the ingredients list on processed foods can give you a rough idea. Here are some tips to help you interpret the information on these labels and determine if a product might be high or low in FODMAPs:

- **Ingredients are listed by weight**, from highest to lowest. So, if high-FODMAP ingredients are among the first few listed, the product is likely high in FODMAPs.
- Even if the ingredients listed are low in FODMAPs, the product might still contain high FODMAP levels due to processing methods or serving size.
- If you're unsure about the FODMAP content, try a small portion when your symptoms are under control and monitor how you feel. If you tolerate it well, it's generally safe to include it in your diet.
- **Gluten-free doesn't always mean low-FODMAP**. Always check for high-FODMAP ingredients like garlic, onion, dried fruits, and fruit juices.
- Many dips and sauces contain added garlic and/or onion, so check carefully.

Common High-FODMAP Ingredients to Watch For

If any of the following are listed among the first few ingredients, it could mean the product is high in FODMAPs.

Fructose:
- High-fructose corn syrup
- Honey
- Fruit juice or fruit juice concentrate (like apple or pear)
- Crystalline fructose
- Agave syrup
- Dried fruit

Polyols:
- Sorbitol
- Mannitol
- Xylitol
- Isomalt
- Erythritol
- Prune juice

Fructans:
- Garlic (including garlic salt, powder, or extract)
- Onion (including onion salt, powder, or extract)
- Wheat, rye, or barley (when listed as a main ingredient)
- Inulin (often added as fiber or prebiotic)
- Chicory root and chicory root extract
- Fructooligosaccharides (FOS).

Carefully reading labels and being aware of these ingredients can help you make more informed choices on a low-FODMAP diet.

Dining Out on a Low-FODMAP Diet

Eating out while following a low-FODMAP diet can be challenging, as high-FODMAP ingredients like garlic and onion are common in restaurant dishes but often aren't listed on menus. Unlike the gluten-free diet, the low-FODMAP diet may not be well understood by restaurant staff, so you may need to spend a little time explaining your dietary needs to the waitstaff or kitchen staff. Here are some tips to help you navigate dining out and enjoy a variety of cuisines while sticking to your diet:

- **Check menus online** ahead of time for restaurants or cafes with potential low-FODMAP options.
- **Identify your key trigger foods** and make sure to ask for them to be left out of your meal.
- Order gluten-free dishes that also avoid your biggest trigger ingredients.
- Opt for **protein-based dishes** like fish, red meat, or poultry served with sides such as vegetables, salads, potatoes, rice, or rice noodles instead of bread or pasta.

Chapter 6: Practical Tips and Recommendations

- Avoid dishes that are heavily sauced or rich (like curries), as these are often difficult to modify and frequently contain garlic and onion.
- Be cautious with soups and risottos, as they often contain stock with garlic and onion.
- Request no garlic or onion, or ask for suggestions on dishes that naturally exclude these ingredients.
- **Ask for sauces, dressings, and dips on the side**, as they often contain garlic and onion.
- **Call ahead** during off-peak hours if you have more complex dietary requests.

Cuisines and Dishes Likely to Have Low-FODMAP Options

Vietnamese:

- Rice vermicelli with beef, chicken, prawn, or tofu (request firm tofu and no onion in the salad)
- Rice paper rolls (ask for no onion)
- Bun dishes (ask for sauces on the side, plain meat if marinated in garlic, and no onion in the salad).

Thai:

- Avoid curries, as they typically contain high-FODMAP ingredients and are harder to modify. Opt for stir-fry dishes with steamed jasmine rice (Khao Plao). Request firm tofu, mild chili, and no garlic or onion. Examples include:
    - Duck breast stir-fry with lemongrass, chili (mild), coriander, and sweet basil
    - Vegetarian stir-fry with firm tofu and low-FODMAP veggies
    - Prawn and mixed seafood stir-fry with capsicum, mild chili, and green beans (Pad Talay).

Japanese:

- Japanese serving sizes are often small, so higher FODMAP ingredients may be tolerable in small amounts, such as avocado in hand rolls or wheat in tempura batter. Soy sauce and wasabi are low-FODMAP. Options include:
    - Sushi, sashimi, and tempura (ask for condiments on the side)
    - Grilled tofu, seafood, beef, or chicken served with rice, vegetables, or seaweed

◆ Rice noodles with your choice of meat and vegetables.

Korean:

- Korean BBQ allows you to select ingredients, so you can build a dish with low-FODMAP items cooked in front of you.

Greek:

- Low-FODMAP options include:
  ◆ Saganaki, plain olives, horta, chargrilled fish, scallops, octopus, tiger prawns, patates, spit-roasted chicken, and mixed grills with salad.
  ◆ Avoid dips, moussaka, pasticcio, and honey-based desserts.

Pub Meals and Pizza:

- Try pizza with a gluten-free crust and low-FODMAP toppings.
- Choose grilled meat, chicken, or fish with steamed veggies, salad, or potato. Request sauces on the side and plain meat if it's marinated.

With a little planning and these tips, you can enjoy eating out while sticking to your low-FODMAP diet!

Traveling on a Low-FODMAP Diet

Many people with IBS worry about managing their symptoms while traveling, as it can be challenging to prepare meals and navigate unfamiliar foods. The change in routine, along with travel and airline meals, can also be a concern. However, a lot of travelers find that their IBS symptoms actually improve while on vacation because stress—a common IBS trigger—is often reduced. Here are some tips to help you stay on track with a low-FODMAP diet while traveling:

- **Complete the re-challenge phase before your trip**, if possible. This way, you'll know which foods are your main triggers and can follow the least restrictive version of the diet while you're away.
- **Learn how to say "no" to certain foods** (like onion and garlic) in the local language to help communicate your needs.
- Airplane meals are usually small, so some high-FODMAP ingredients (like broccoli, beetroot, or butternut squash) may be tolerable in limited quantities.

- **Call the airline in advance** to request a meal that avoids your trigger foods. A gluten-free meal might work but be sure to check for high-FODMAP items like onion, garlic, and fruit juice.
- Bring **low-FODMAP snacks** for the flight, such as nuts and fruits that are safe for your diet.
- Keep any **medications for managing IBS symptoms** in your carry-on, so they're easily accessible.
- Consider **booking self-contained accommodation** with a kitchen so you can prepare some of your own meals.
- Look up menus of local restaurants online to find places that may offer low-FODMAP options.

With a little planning, you can have a smoother, more enjoyable trip while managing your low-FODMAP diet.

30-Day Low-FODMAP Diet Plan For IBS

Day 1

- **Breakfast:** Sweet Potato Pancakes with Raspberries
- **Lunch:** Quinoa Tabbouleh
- **Dinner:** Grilled Shrimp with Lemon and Herbs
- **Snack:** Low-FODMAP Chia Seed Pudding

Total Calories: 1750 kcal

Vitamins:
- Vitamin A 700 mcg
- Vitamin C 90 mg
- Vitamin D 600 IU
- Calcium 900 mg
- Iron 15 mg

Day 2

- **Breakfast:** Carrot Cake Porridge
- **Lunch:** Shrimp Saganaki
- **Dinner:** Mediterranean Baked Cod with Tomatoes and Olives
- **Snack:** Pumpkin Spice Protein Balls

Total Calories: 1800 kcal

Vitamins:
- Vitamin A 800 mcg
- Vitamin C 100 mg
- Calcium 950 mg
- Iron 18 mg

Day 3

- **Breakfast:** Poached Egg Sandwich with Smoked Salmon
- **Lunch:** Grilled Lamb Chops with Mint
- **Dinner:** Zucchini and Ground Turkey Skillet
- **Snack:** Cranberry Orange Protein Balls

Total Calories: 1780 kcal

Vitamins:
- Vitamin A 750 mcg
- Vitamin C 120 mg
- Calcium 800 mg
- Iron 17 mg

Day 4

- **Breakfast:** Vegan French Toast
- **Lunch:** Chicken Piccata
- **Dinner:** One-Skillet Ground Turkey Thai Curry with Rice
- **Snack:** Fig and Date Energy Balls

Total Calories: 1900 kcal

Vitamins:
- Vitamin A 680 mcg
- Vitamin C 85 mg
- Calcium 820 mg
- Iron 19 mg

Day 5

- **Breakfast:** Scrambled Tofu
- **Lunch:** Greek-Style Meatballs
- **Dinner:** Mediterranean Salmon with Caper Relish
- **Snack:** Mixed Berry & Yogurt Granola Bar

Total Calories: 1720 kcal

Vitamins:
- Vitamin A 820 mcg
- Vitamin C 95 mg
- Calcium 930 mg
- Iron 16 mg

Day 6

- **Breakfast:** Coconut Blueberry Smoothie
- **Lunch:** Low-FODMAP Japanese Chicken Katsu
- **Dinner:** Turkey Stuffed Bell Peppers
- **Snack:** Salted Caramel Peanut Candy Bars

Total Calories: 1850 kcal

Vitamins:
- Vitamin A 710 mcg
- Vitamin C 70 mg
- Calcium 880 mg
- Iron 15 mg

Day 7

- **Breakfast:** Tropical Millet Porridge
- **Lunch:** Beef Burger with Lactose-Free Cheese
- **Dinner:** Shredded Brussels Sprout Salad with Roasted Sweet Potatoes
- **Snack:** Peanut Butter Energy Bars

Total Calories: 1700 kcal

Vitamins:
- Vitamin A 780 mcg
- Vitamin C 100 mg
- Calcium 950 mg
- Iron 18 mg

Day 8

- **Breakfast:** Huevos Rancheros Hummus Toast
- **Lunch:** Asian-Inspired Quinoa Salad
- **Dinner:** Lemon Herb Turkey Cutlets with Roasted Vegetables
- **Snack:** Savory Muffin

Total Calories: 1750 kcal

Vitamins:
- Vitamin A 740 mcg
- Vitamin C 120 mg
- Calcium 870 mg
- Iron 16 mg

Day 9

- **Breakfast:** Chia Seed Pudding
- **Lunch:** Chicken Avocado Burger
- **Dinner:** Garlic-Infused Olive Oil Shrimp and Spinach Sauté
- **Snack:** Spiced Molasses Cookies

Total Calories: 1800 kcal

Vitamins:
- Vitamin A 800 mcg
- Vitamin C 90 mg
- Calcium 920 mg
- Iron 17 mg

Day 10

- **Breakfast:** Baked Sweet Potatoes with Almond Butter
- **Lunch:** Salmon with Dill and Lemon
- **Dinner:** Mongolian Turkey
- **Snack:** Pumpkin Spice Protein Balls

Total Calories: 1780 kcal

Vitamins:
- Vitamin A 700 mcg
- Vitamin C 110 mg
- Calcium 880 mg
- Iron 15 mg

Day 11

- **Breakfast:** Gluten-Free Waffles with Strawberries
- **Lunch:** Warm Chicken and Roast Vegetable Salad
- **Dinner:** Beef and Tomato Stir-Fry with Fresh Basil
- **Snack:** Peanut Butter and Hemp Seed Protein Balls

Total Calories: 1850 kcal

Vitamins:
- Vitamin A 770 mcg
- Vitamin C 95 mg
- Calcium 930 mg
- Iron 18 mg

Day 12

- **Breakfast:** Protein Overnight Oats
- **Lunch:** Turkey Burger with Spinach
- **Dinner:** Creamy Vegan Mushroom Soup
- **Snack:** Cranberry Orange Protein Balls

Total Calories: 1800 kcal

Vitamins:
- Vitamin A 760 mcg
- Vitamin C 100 mg
- Calcium 890 mg
- Iron 19 mg

Day 13

- **Breakfast:** Peach and Raspberry Smoothie
- **Lunch:** Tandoori Chicken
- **Dinner:** Turkey Meatballs with Tomato Basil Sauce
- **Snack:** Mixed Berry & Yogurt Granola Bar

Total Calories: 1750 kcal

Vitamins:
- Vitamin A 820 mcg
- Vitamin C 80 mg
- Calcium 850 mg
- Iron 16 mg

Day 14

- **Breakfast:** Spinach, Feta & Pine Nut Omelet
- **Lunch:** Pork Lettuce Wraps
- **Dinner:** Shakshuka
- **Snack:** Fig and Date Energy Balls

Total Calories: 1820 kcal

Vitamins:
- Vitamin A 700 mcg
- Vitamin C 90 mg
- Calcium 930 mg
- Iron 17 mg

Day 15

- **Breakfast:** Quinoa Porridge with Banana & Yogurt
- **Lunch:** Mediterranean Chicken Skewers
- **Dinner:** Orange Ginger Grilled Chicken
- **Snack:** Salted Caramel Peanut Candy Bars

Total Calories: 1800 kcal

Vitamins:
Vitamin A 720 mcg
Vitamin C 95 mg
Calcium 870 mg
Iron 18 mg

Day 16

- **Breakfast:** Scrambled Tofu
- **Lunch:** Low-FODMAP Vietnamese Pho
- **Dinner:** Basil Coconut Milk Ground Beef Skillet
- **Snack:** Peanut Butter Energy Bars

Total Calories: 1850 kcal

Vitamins:
- Vitamin A 770 mcg
- Vitamin C 100 mg
- Calcium 920 mg
- Iron 16 mg

Day 17

- **Breakfast:** Sweet Potato Pancakes with Raspberries
- **Lunch:** Shrimp Saganaki
- **Dinner:** Turkey Patties with Olive Tapenade
- **Snack:** Pumpkin Spice Protein Balls

Total Calories: 1750 kcal

Chapter 6: Practical Tips and Recommendations

Vitamins:
- Vitamin A 800 mcg
- Vitamin C 110 mg
- Calcium 900 mg
- Iron 15 mg

Day 18

- **Breakfast:** Vegan French Toast
- **Lunch:** Beef Burger with Lactose-Free Cheese
- **Dinner:** Zucchini and Ground Turkey Skillet
- **Snack:** Spiced Molasses Cookies

Total Calories: 1800 kcal

Vitamins:
- Vitamin A 680 mcg
- Vitamin C 95 mg
- Calcium 930 mg
- Iron 17 mg

Day 19

- **Breakfast:** Coconut Lime Smoothie
- **Lunch:** Asian-Inspired Quinoa Salad
- **Dinner:** Chicken and Gnocchi Casserole
- **Snack:** Peanut Butter and Hemp Seed Protein Balls

Total Calories: 1780 kcal

Vitamins:
- Vitamin A 740 mcg
- Vitamin C 100 mg
- Calcium 870 mg
- Iron 16 mg

Day 20

- **Breakfast:** Chia Seed Pudding
- **Lunch:** Grilled Lamb Chops with Mint
- **Dinner:** Salmon Bowls with Avocado and Carrot "Rice"
- **Snack:** Cranberry Orange Protein Balls

Total Calories: 1800 kcal

Vitamins:
- Vitamin A 800 mcg
- Vitamin C 90 mg
- Calcium 930 mg
- Iron 18 mg

Day 21

- **Breakfast:** Tropical Millet Porridge
- **Lunch:** Chicken Avocado Burger
- **Dinner:** Mediterranean Baked Cod with Tomatoes and Olives
- **Snack:** Fig and Date Energy Balls

Total Calories: 1750 kcal

Vitamins:
- Vitamin A 780 mcg
- Vitamin C 85 mg
- Calcium 890 mg
- Iron 15 mg

Day 22

- **Breakfast:** Peach and Raspberry Smoothie
- **Lunch:** Greek-Style Meatballs
- **Dinner:** Mongolian Turkey
- **Snack:** Mixed Berry & Yogurt Granola Bar

Total Calories: 1850 kcal

Vitamins:
- Vitamin A 820 mcg
- Vitamin C 120 mg
- Calcium 900 mg
- Iron 16 mg

Day 23

- **Breakfast:** Spinach, Feta & Pine Nut Omelet
- **Lunch:** Mediterranean Chicken Skewers
- **Dinner:** Turkey Stuffed Bell Peppers
- **Snack:** Pumpkin Spice Protein Balls

Total Calories: 1820 kcal

Vitamins:
- Vitamin A 700 mcg
- Vitamin C 90 mg
- Calcium 880 mg
- Iron 15 mg

Day 24

- **Breakfast:** Quinoa Porridge with Banana & Yogurt
- **Lunch:** Chicken Piccata
- **Dinner:** Shredded Brussels Sprout Salad with Roasted Sweet Potatoes
- **Snack:** Peanut Butter Energy Bars

Total Calories: 1750 kcal

Vitamins:
- Vitamin A 760 mcg
- Vitamin C 100 mg
- Calcium 910 mg
- Iron 16 mg

Day 25

- **Breakfast:** Sweet Potato Pancakes with Raspberries
- **Lunch:** Shrimp Saganaki
- **Dinner:** Garlic-Infused Olive Oil Shrimp and Spinach Sauté
- **Snack:** Fig and Date Energy Balls

Total Calories: 1780 kcal

Vitamins:
- Vitamin A 700 mcg
- Vitamin C 85 mg
- Calcium 880 mg
- Iron 17 mg

Day 26

- **Breakfast:** Vegan French Toast
- **Lunch:** Warm Chicken and Roast Vegetable Salad
- **Dinner:** Orange Ginger Grilled Chicken
- **Snack:** Cranberry Orange Protein Balls

Total Calories: 1800 kcal

Vitamins:
- Vitamin A 800 mcg
- Vitamin C 100 mg
- Calcium 900 mg
- Iron 15 mg

Day 27

- **Breakfast:** Scrambled Tofu
- **Lunch:** Low-FODMAP Vietnamese Pho
- **Dinner:** Mediterranean Salmon with Caper Relish
- **Snack:** Mixed Berry & Yogurt Granola Bar

Total Calories: 1750 kcal

Vitamins:
- Vitamin A 780 mcg
- Vitamin C 90 mg
- Calcium 850 mg
- Iron 18 mg

Day 28

- **Breakfast:** Peach and Raspberry Smoothie
- **Lunch:** Asian-Inspired Quinoa Salad
- **Dinner:** Spiced Beef Patties with Cucumber Yogurt Sauce
- **Snack:** Pumpkin Spice Protein Balls

Total Calories: 1850 kcal

Vitamins:
- Vitamin A 700 mcg
- Vitamin C 85 mg
- Calcium 930 mg
- Iron 16 mg

Day 29

- **Breakfast:** Tropical Millet Porridge
- **Lunch:** Greek-Style Meatballs
- **Dinner:** Creamy Vegan Mushroom Soup
- **Snack:** Salted Caramel Peanut Candy Bars

Total Calories: 1800 kcal

Vitamins:
- Vitamin A 720 mcg
- Vitamin C 100 mg
- Calcium 900 mg
- Iron 17 mg

Day 30

- **Breakfast:** Protein Overnight Oats
- **Lunch:** Chicken Avocado Burger
- **Dinner:** Mediterranean Baked Cod with Tomatoes and Olives
- **Snack:** Fig and Date Energy Balls

Total Calories: 1750 kcal

Vitamins:
- Vitamin A 760 mcg
- Vitamin C 95 mg
- Calcium 920 mg
- Iron 18 mg

Each person requires a different amount of calories based on their lifestyle. For example, individuals with an active lifestyle need more energy compared to those with a sedentary lifestyle. This meal plan is provided for informational purposes, and you can supplement it with the recommended side dishes to meet your specific calorie needs.

In today's fast-paced world, we often find ourselves too busy to cook three different meals every single day. However, that doesn't mean you can't stick to a healthy eating plan like this 30-day Low-FODMAP diet. One simple solution is to select a day, such as Day 1, and prepare enough food to last for 2-3 days.

This approach not only helps you stick to the plan but also allows you to enjoy variety without the daily pressure of cooking multiple dishes. Prepping in advance ensures you stay on track with your nutritional goals, even on your busiest days.

Made in the USA
Las Vegas, NV
06 February 2025

17677816R00066